Book Recommendations

I0039436

Dr. Inez Cotton has made a valuable contribution to the ministries of the Church by focusing our attention on "antepartum mothers." It is rare to find churches who see this as a need. Hospital chaplains cannot carry this burden alone. Dr. Cotton provides the needed information for sensitizing us to this valuable ministry.

Dr. Emmanuel L. McCall
Retired pastor and seminary professor, popular lecturer
Atlanta, Georgia

Dr. Inez Cotton has carefully captured the learnings from her Doctor of Ministry Project on pastoral care and ministry among antepartum mothers. She provides keen insight, personal anecdotes, and theological and biblical understanding to the ministry of caring before childbirth. This is a timely word for the church and every follower of Jesus who aims to stand with pregnant mothers in distress, in the joys, and challenges of childbirth.

Albert L. Reyes, D.Min, PhD
President and CEO
Buckner International

"Dr. Cotton gives both heart and attention to women needing extra tender loving care during possible traumatic life altering events they might experience before childbirth. Her training and call to serve them make her one of the leading champions on this subject. The church is being called upon to embrace this matter and shepherd families through an event that can open the door for congregants to experience ministry like never before."

Michael A. Evans, D Min.,
Pastor, Texas Baptist Denominational Leader, Civic and Community Servant

Triumphant Hope in the Midst of Despair: Supporting Antepartum Mothers

Inez B. Cotton

Terry Austin, Editor

Copyright @ 2020 by Inez Goldie Barge Cotton

All Rights Reserved

Published by Austin Brothers Publishing, Fort Worth, Texas

www.abpbooks.com

Front cover image by Katie Reinhart

ISBN 978-1-7333130-2-5

Library of Congress Control Number: 2020901151

Copyright © 2020 by Inez Cotton

ALL RIGHTS RESERVED. *No part of this book may be reproduced in any form without permission in writing from the publisher, except in the case of brief quotations embodied in critical reviews or articles.*

Printed in the United States of America

2020 -- First Edition

DEDICATION

Gratitude to my husband, R. J., whose love, prayers, spiritual, and donor support kept me focused throughout this spiritual journey. I am also grateful for his positive and godly energy that kept my faith and focus on God the Father, God the Son, and God the Holy Spirit. Gratitude to Roy's brothers, X. L. Cotton (Georgia, posthumously), and Palmer L. Cotton (Joyce); for their tangible and spiritual support, as they modeled for us the virtues of marriage and family. Gratitude to the rest of R. J.'s family who have caused me to feel at home in a distant land.

Gratitude to my sons and their spouses, Jay (Niya) and Justin (Carolina), for their personhood, faith, college institutions, and vocations that helped them find true love and marital bliss. Our sons' flexibility was appreciated amidst my educational and vocational pursuits during their high school and early college years.

Gratitude to my grandchildren, Roy III, Eric, and Nyla, who kept me grounded with their natural humor and unconditional love for me. Each one helped me balance this project with a continuous focus on the family.

Gratitude to my siblings, their spouses, and their children; Jacqueline Reeves (Robert), Estelle Langston, Jean Gentry (posthumously), Bernice Phillips, John Barge, Jr., (posthumously), and Jean (sister-in-law), Evangeline Hasket (Bill), and Jessie Laughton; for being my educational and experiential mentors, and for their continuous and loving support of me throughout this project.

Gratitude to the memory of my parents, John and Willie Barge, who invested in me in more ways than I can articulate as they modeled the virtues of hard work, kind Christian living, and their enduring diligence in raising eight children.

Gratitude to Dr. Larry Ashlock, whose scholarly inquiries and theological suggestions broadened the scope of this project. Gratitude to Dr. Margaret Lawson, my supervisor, who helped me maintain high educational curriculum standards in this paper. Gratitude to Michel Mullender, the Baylor Hospital Pastoral Care Director (Baylor University Medical Center/ Dallas Area Hospitals) for serving on the Doctoral Programs Council.

Gratitude to the supportive Baylor Scott & White Office of Mission and Ministry (BSWH), R. Mark Grace, Vice President and Chief Missions and Ministry Officer; Baylor University Medical Center Staff, Michel Mullender, Director/ Dallas Area Hospitals; Millicent Albert, Pastoral Care Manager; Kayla Carey, Manager of the Neonatal Intensive Care Unit (NICU), and Kristine Debuty, Director, Maternal Child Health. Clinical Pastoral Education (CPE), Carlos Bell, Director; Lauren Frazier McGuin, Certified Educator; and the 7 Jonsson Staff, for providing patients for this project, and to the amazing Chaplain Residents participation in the project. Gratitude to Sherry Shanks and Clay Price for their assistance in calibrating and structuring the on-line surveys.

Gratitude to Terry Austin for editing this book and for the great professional support rendered by the Austin Brothers Publishing Company.

Gratitude to all of my chaplain colleagues, all on the Baylor healthcare team, and all of the encouraging individuals named and unnamed, who helped me stay focused on this project.

Contents

Preface

If you're interested in learning about 21st Century understanding of early pregnancies, I am grateful that you picked up this book. You will be introduced to a term that might be new to you— "antepartum." It is the opposite of postpartum (meaning after childbirth). Antepartum addresses pre-birth. This book is an extension of my doctoral thesis completed during my time serving as a chaplain at Baylor Hospital in Dallas. I am now retired after enjoying the daily task of serving as a staff chaplain in Women and Children's Services in the area of Maternal Child Health, at Baylor Hospital in Dallas.

God has blessed me to write about antepartum mothers. These experiences have become near and dear to me. I deeply enjoyed Baylor, and this book will also detail much from my doctoral project as a student at B.H. Carroll Institute in Irving, TX. My goal for this book is to provide spiritual support to all who want to explore the intriguing world of mothers-to-be inside and outside of the hospital setting. It is my hope that after you read the contents of this book, you find comfort in what you already know about expectant mothers and also discover new ways to support family, friends, and other women who find themselves anticipating birth.

I will also provide suggestions on how to engage normal as well as at-risk pre-term mothers who are content, scared, worried, or lacking throughout their antepartum experiences. My prayer is that you join the ranks of those who make concerted efforts to support and listen to the needs of all expectant mothers. I seek to present and prepare others to practice and address the unspoken concerns of women who want to hear a word from the Creator God. Our hands and feet can administer warmth and hope that is ordained by a loving God.

The project began by leading seven student chaplains to look at five themes (see Chapter Three), in my quest to help pregnant women cope with the blessings and challenges while on hospital bed rest. The study aimed to address the levels of spiritual distress in the women over a six-week period. At the end of the project, we discovered from the statistical tool, that spiritual support for the mothers-to-be was varied, case by case. To make it understandable, the findings produced no formal conclusion on how to address all pregnant women's spiritual challenges. Each experience is her own and distinct to her personal and medical situation. The findings, listed after the study, brought value about personal and professional relationships that had a life of their own.

Significant for me in the preparation phase of this project was my initial call and subsequent preparation as a church worker, hospital chaplain, my role as a wife, daughter, parent, and grandparent. I was licensed and ordained in the gospel ministry in Virginia. I am endorsed by the Baptist General Convention (Texas Baptists), and a board certified Chaplain with the Association of Professional Chaplains. Life experience, chaplaincy training, seminary training, church and family experiences, my former time as an art teacher in Norfolk, VA, provided a rich foundation as I experienced the challenges in this project. My teaching experience provided a surprise connection to this book. The number of teen pregnancies and other unwed mothers at an alternative school helped align similar story lines in both venues.

The gist of the book centers on how I studied and supported these women theologically. You, the reader, may want to start with these themes and then look at the rest of my findings. Chapter 3 details five themes included in the original doctoral paper for B.H. Carroll Theological Institute in Irving, TX, in 2019. B.H. Carroll houses a group of dedicated theologians, professors, and educators who have an interest in providing local and global theological education to the masses. Baylor Hospital is an amazing healthcare institution with professionals and chaplains who reflect a holistic approach to quality healthcare to faith-based as well as non-faith-based patients. These two institutions helped me live out this dream. For this I am grateful.

This book is written from a Christian perspective. The contents include practical approaches to professional healthcare to antepartum or pre-term hospital patients. The seven chaplain residents and I determined whether the patient's level of spiritual distress could be significantly helped by the hospital chaplains ministry. We sought to support them the best way possible with the available resources we had in ourselves and the wide range of professional support around us. The course of a single life from beginning to end developes with a consistency of empathetic care. We sought to figure out how best to spiritually support women who seldom initiated chaplain visitation.

The conclusion of this study is significant. The report is conclusive to the life of a patient. A larger than life presence of family, church, community, chaplains, and others on the healthcare team help the mother cope with at-risk pregnancies.

The photographs in this book chronicle my life story. My mothers' antepartum experiences branched out from the support she received when she carried me. Now I have my personal antepartum story. The stages of all antepartum stories are likewise unique to everyone's journey. The Spiritual Journey genogram invites all to consider the powerful gift of relationship. A genogram gives mothers-to-be the opportunity to cite people and institutions that have contributed to their autobiographical history. The antepartum journey branches out to others as our Triune God nurtures patients. The photographs serve as a pictorial spiritual journey genogram found in the appendix. I encourage each reader to see a broader spiritual picture for each antepartum mother they encounter. The theological themes may serve you to amply see each mother-to-be.

The goal of this book is to assist all helpers who have entered this intriguing world. I am grateful to all of the Baylor Maternal Child Health Staff (MCH), the Office of Mission and Ministry Staff at Baylor (OMM), the seven Jonsson staff, the seven students who were my supporters in the project. I am also grateful for the wonderful patients, families, and the Baylor Hospital staff who allowed me and other chaplains to enter the antepartum world.

The photographs serve as a pictorial spiritual journey genogram located at the end of this book. The pictures tell my story, demonstrating what the chaplain residents presented to patients in the form of diagrams. The patients were asked to highlight pivotal people, places, and other supportive venues in their life journeys. We learned from this exercise that we too could model and benefit from detailing the snippets of our own narratives that conclusively helped us cope in times of despair. The reader is encouraged likewise to recall great memories in one's life journey. Accentuating the positive aids in coping skills during stressful times.

Foreword

This project began as a study on spiritual distress or a broad definition of stress in hospital antepartum or pregnant patients. The primary approach was to study the significance of receiving pastoral support from chaplains and others. This study also addresses the unique processes and useful descriptions of the work needed and practiced by supportive families and communities, professional chaplains, chaplain residents (participants in the project), theologians, and other hospital healthcare providers. The plan evolved into a six-week course for chaplain residents, facilitated by a staff chaplain, my role in the project.

After this study, I envision a renewed list of empathizers for antepartum women. There is a need for more support for these women and their families, from church and community institutions, mid-wives, families, and friends. The study sought to determine the significance of the spiritual dimension of care for the antepatum patients. The hope was to identify a renewed family mode of support, theological emphases, and on-point ministerial perspectives about pastoral care of antepartum patients. Are these mothers experiencing vast levels of spiritual distress, and if so, what pastoral or other human support is needed to assist them in the midst of patients and family crucial circumstances?

We also sought to determine if there could be significance in identifying spiritual distress in antepartum patients at Baylor Medical Center in Dallas, Texas. We also wanted to discover whether there were other claims or aspects of spiritual distress that might support or deny spiritual awarenesses described in this project. Other questions might address: What might supporters of pre-term mothers best consider or discover as they address spiritual distress in prenatal mothers? Are the theological themes in this paper significant enough to address the vast spiritual needs of the twenty-first-century mother-to-be? Lastly, what antepartum community groups or demographics may need to be addressed (i.e., older women, career women, sexual abuse, human trafficking, adoption, foster care [advanced child protective services], surrogacy, or other current culture trends)?

In conclusion, we ask, will the theological themes in this project provide a level of comfort for patients experiencing spiritual distress inside or outside of the hospital? Are there other theological themes that should be added to the listed topics (The Image of God, God and Suffering, Jesus, The Suffering Servant, Eschatological Hope, and The Church.)?

Introduction

This book and all the people involved in its creation present a formidable foundation for learning and growth. I hope you will find Chapter 3 especially useful as blessings from a loving Creator and a list of five theological themes which provide theological perspectives for providers and families. New lives are about to be welcomed into many family systems or other teams of support. My interest in antepartum, pregnant, or pre-term labor patients and their families developed through a series of personal, vocational, church, and family life experiences.[1] I have learned first-hand the importance of family and spiritual support when a woman awaits the birth of a baby.

In my own past, Christian faith helped me and my husband Roy come to terms with an undetermined pre-term medical condition that our family physician discovered early in pregnancy. I experienced a daunting level of stress related to the unknown, exacerbated by the wait before a prognosis could be determined. The experience was unsettling for both of us. As a stay-at-home mother, at the time,

---

1 See chapter 5, "Implications for Contemporary Ministry and the Project Director's Early Ministry Connections that Highlight the Project Director's Vocational, Church, and Family History."

we had the additional challenge of caring for our toddler son with no other family members living in the city.

Waiting for the unknown was challenging, especially when the doctor suggested the possibility of problems before childbirth because of my age. Later, to our surprise and joy, the physician informed us the good news that the baby's perceived problems were nonexistent.

Before retirement as a Baylor hospital chaplain, I remember countless other prenatal stories in my own history with family members who reported undetermined prognoses of their unborn babies. The additional family history would help me to connect with antepartum patients at Baylor Scott and White Health in Dallas, TX. As stated in the dedication, my heartfelt gratitude is expressed to R. Mark Grace, Mike Mullender, Millicent Albert, the seven Jonsson staff, The Women and Children's staff at Baylor, the Chaplain Residents and the Clinical Pastoral Education Department with Carlos Bell and Lauren Frazier-McGuin.

Ministry to Pregnant Women - a Chaplain's Perspective

learned many helpful skills as a chaplain about antepartum or pregnant patients during my earlier internship at Baylor University Medical Center in Dallas. The Clinical Pastoral Education program (CPE) began for me in the summer of 2005 at Baylor University Medical Center in Dallas. The Clinical Pastoral Education classes included Interpersonal Relations (IPR), individual and group supervision, and an overall introduction to CPE. The Theological Integration classes helped me look theologically at situations during patient visitations. I was introduced to Maternal Child Health (MCH) during my first clinical assignment as a CPE intern.[2] David Hormenoo was the student supervisor in the Clinical Pastoral Education Program at that time, under the leadership of Mark Grace who was then the Association of Clinical Pastoral Care Supervisor and Director of Baylor's Department of Pastoral Care and Counseling across North Dallas and Central Texas.

---

2 I began the Clinical Pastoral Education Program (CPE) during a summer intensive program at Baylor University Medical Center in Dallas, Texas, in 2005. I also provided patient care to the Baylor Institute of Rehabilitation during the summer intensive unit.

The beginning summer internship was challenging. As an intern fresh out of seminary (2004, Southwestern Baptist Theological Seminary in Fort Worth, TX), I recall shadowing the MCH chaplain on several visits. I learned first-hand the importance of assessing the needs of patients before providing spiritual support. The need for empathetic listening, attending skills, and supportive dialogue was demonstrated during those times. Patients responded well to the compassionate dialogue with the staff chaplain, Ella McCarroll. Noticeable was reframing the identical comments made by each patient as they spoke to the chaplain. Affirmations and supportive dialogue seemed to match and highlight what the patients expressed. This was renewed insight for me as we worked through the Clinical Pastoral Education compentencies in class.

The antepartum patients are located at the Baylor Medical Center in Dallas (BUMC) on the seventh floor of the Jonsson Building. As stated earlier, the preliminary introduction to these patients contributed to my interest in this project. Divine call, ongoing seminary training, and spiritual interest in Maternal Child Health (MCH) were other contributing factors.[3] The didactics, the Interpersonal Relations classes (IPR), individual and group supervision, the theological

---

3 The clinical coordinators during summer internship were Ella McCarroll in MCH and Melissa Walker-Luckett at BIR (summer of 2005). Other history includes; full-time Chaplain I Resident at the North Texas Veterans' Affairs Hospital in Dallas (2005-06), and a second year of residency at Baylor, Dallas, from 2007 to 2008. I served in "Fellow" Chaplain Resident II (including a second year of residency at BUMC), and PRN positions until 2009. The project director's earlier and related Clinical Pastoral Education history as a chaplain were: PRN service at the Baylor Institute of Rehabilitation (BIR) at Baylor Medical Center in Dallas (BUMC). CenterPointe Baptist Church in Red Oak, Texas, is the location of my volunteer ministry as Christian educator (my husband was the founder of CenterPointe Baptist Church). From July 2013 to July 2016, I was employed at BUMC as a Chaplain Resident II Fellow in MCH, funded by the Chilton Foundation. I was recently promoted (July 2016) to Staff Chaplain II in Women and Children's Services (W&CS). Millicent Albert, supervisor and a Pastoral Care Manager at BUMC. My husband (Roy) and I are currently members of Singing Hills Baptist Church, where I have served as a grief counselor and also as a coach in Children's Church.

integration classes, and the overall introduction to CPE were beneficial to my pastoral education training.

Many other learning opportunities prepared me for chaplaincy
after my initial internship. The additional completion of four units
of CPE at the North Texas Veterans Affairs Hospital in Dallas broadened the scope of my training.[4] Later I was invited back to Baylor
to serve as a PRN, several other chaplain fellow positions, and was
accepted to complete four more units in the second year of residency. Additional service lines were also explored in these positions at
Baylor. I looked forward to calls that requested pastoral care providers to visit labor-and-delivery patients. The opportunity transitioned
again for me to return as a stay-at-home mother (for four years) and
later completed more seminary training at B. H. Carroll Theological
Institute, then in Arlington, Texas. Recently, I completed APC Board
Certification and then served as the Maternal Child Health Staff
Chaplain in Women and Children's services. These professional,
ministerial, and family experiences contributed to the development
of this project.

The new leadership position provided opportunities for me to
address antepartum patients' needs in a renewed light. I began to
internally ask myself a series of questions about how I would provide heartfelt spiritual and pastoral support to patients. I asked, "Am
I providing adequate care to antepartum patients?" Another issue
was, "What other spiritual factors are needed to ensure the utmost
support of prenatal women?"

From these internal inquiries grew in me a deep desire to better connect to the hospital antepartum patient. The on-going

---

4 The essential training at the Veteran Affairs Hospital in Dallas enhanced
the training in preparation for my return to Baylor Hospital. The first complete
first-year residency in the project director's CPE training was at the North Texas
Veterans Affairs Hospital (VA) in Dallas, Texas. My supervisors were Joe Gross
(Early founder and champion for the CPE program at Baylor Hospitals, Retired)
and JoAnn Garma (Retired).

development of the project would present a broader inquiry for the chaplain. My role was expanded, as now I would lead chaplain residents, chaplain PRN's, chaplain interns, and other members of the healthcare team on 7J who would help me with my concerns. They would now look to the chaplain for clinical coordination and spiritual guidance. Therefore, the larger question for this study is, "How might chaplains improve their pastoral care of antepartum patients who are experiencing spiritual distress in the hospital setting?" I would also have the resource of Millicent Albert who formerly served in my role but moved to a Pastoral Care Manager position.

With the help of my B. H. Carroll Theological Institute professors, I presented a research study regarding, "the significance of pastoral care in addressing spiritual distress in antepartum patients at Baylor Scott and White Health at Dallas Area Hospitals," the title of my project.

A pre-term mother's stay in the hospital might last for an indefinite period. Extreme medical problems might revolve around a mother's prognosis, and/or the medical needs of her growing baby. The delicate nature of a baby's medical issues during gestational growth might cause challenges for the patient's family, friends, other support systems, and/or employers. This project introduced a level of spiritual baggage for patients. Mother-to-be might carry complex medical needs. Some prognoses may lean toward human interdependence and survival between mothers and babies. One example follows.

A pre-term mother (S.J) was presented in the ICU with Marfan Syndrome. The parents faced an at-risk pregnancy because of other medical complications. The mother also had an aortic aneurysm. To the surprise of the couple, they were now expecting girl and boy fraternal twins.[5] The Baylor House Supervisor and other Baylor

5 This case is presented by permission from the antepartum mother. A communication board was used to support the antepartum pre-term patient.

upper-level management healthcare providers were on alert that the lives of both the mother and the babies were at risk because of the gravity of the prognosis. For several days, the mother was given medications to sedate and calm her after her emergency surgery at the Heart and Vascular Hospital. Decisions would have to be made about the life of the twins as well as the life of the mother, if or when more complications arose. I visited the patient and family to support the antepartum mother after she was transported to an ICU unit.

The initial visit with the mother was heartwarming. The patient could not talk because she had been intubated. The patient's fraternal twin brother was visiting his sister at the time of this visit. The patient's adult twin brother was ever-present night and day. The couple's home was in a distant Texas county, and the husband managed to visit the patient regularly. During a late evening visit, the twin brother informed me that the patient welcomed faith-based spiritual support, prayer, and/or hymn singing. The patient's responses were inaudible, but the patient's eye expressions seemed to connect with me throughout the initial visit.

Upon my arrival to the Intensive Care Unit (ICU), a telling moment for me occurred after praying and consoling the patient and her twin brother. The mother managed to express a connecting response using her eyes to communicate. I asked the patient whether she wanted continued prayer for herself and her twins. I assessed her emphatic reaction as a "Yes!" Later I would provide a "Communication Board," supplied by the OMM pastoral care office, to communicate secular and spiritual words and phrases that help patients express themselves to others. Later, both the husband and the twin brother of the mother-to-be used the board to help them

Joel Burning (Chaplain). *Spiritual Care Board by Vidatak: An Innovation in Patient Communication* (New York: The New York and Presbyterian Hospital 2013, 2016). The board is a visual guide intended to reduce distress in mechanically ventilated intensive care unit patients. Annal AM Thoracic Soc 2016: 13:1333-1342.

communicate with her. The antepartum mother later reported to others that the chaplain's ministry helped her as she and her family experienced this critical medical event. She eventually delivered her babies and was well on her way to recovery. This is one example among many that highlight the countless complications that can spiritually affect a prenatal mother's state of being in the hospital.

Other antepartum mothers might experience spiritual and physical burdens manifested by loss of control in decision-making and the sudden call for mandatory hospital bedrest. Antepartum patients' compliance with bed rest might warrant instant separation from children, jobs, and in some instances, even one's home state or country. Other spiritual issues may cause the mother to focus on the survival of her baby. She may ask herself how her hospital length-of-stay might affect her family, spouse, or place of employment. The patient may be faced with ongoing financial needs at home, including aging parents and other sick children. An antepartum mother with expressed faith spends much time in prayer over her baby's health and the issues surrounding her illness. Her tensions may stem from a pre-term history of such things as unhealthy eating, poor lifestyle habits, or the patient's perceived mistakes from her past. These thoughts cause some patients to feel they have placed their growing babies at risk.

Several things must be considered when visiting antepartum patients. The chaplain's task is to listen to the needs of patients. Pastors, family members, church members, and others also contribute to the emotional and spiritual welfare of patients. All must check for imbedded biases that might hinder a successful visit. The timing of a visit is important. A patient who has just returned from an in-hospital medical appointment or is being visited during rest time might not welcome visitation. Low lighting may perhaps serve as a clue to the patient's demeanor. A dim room, for instance, may be an attempt to deter visitors. Some patients gladly welcome pastoral visitations and ask the chaplain to turn the light on for them. Many patients may want spiritual support through visitations well in advance of physician visits or problematic social work appointments. Visitations are better welcomed at the patient's or nurse's request. Many doctors request pastoral referrals when they think a visit will support the well-being of their patients. Prenatal mothers tend to enjoy showing off sonogram pictures to family members and staff. An element of joy permeates the room when a sonogram is shown. At this time patients express their joy because all can see that the patient's baby is thriving in spite of medical conditions.

Scheduled induction times or due dates are events that are often celebrated by patients. Prenatal patients also welcome the good news about improved medical prognoses from their physicians. Patients seem overjoyed when they receive permission by their physicians to return home until their due dates. Some patients prefer solitude, while others welcome strong faith-based interactions. Most patients seem to welcome weekly/monthly encouragement flyers, baby blankets, pillows, stuffed animals, and other gestures of support provided by chaplains. Patients enjoy receiving visits from their church pastor and fellow church members. Sensitivity to the length of stay is desired. Good visitations in the eye of patients are ones that lift her spirits or listen well to her concerns. Providers must work hard to give patients permission to feel what they feel. Many feel supported when supporters choose to walk with them.

Many patients welcomed prayer and bible reading by personal request. Patients report that they enjoy the many activities offered to them from hospital and community services. One community service includes, the "Helping Hands Ministry" that supports women who have their physician's permission to sit for one half hour in a meeting setting. The patients participate in crafts and other hands-on activities. In the hospital, several Baylor "in-house" activities also include short wheelchair trips to the four Baylor restaurants or visitations to the three gift shops around the campus. Chaplains provide flyers that inform patients about these activities. Other resources include pet, music, and art therapy,[6] dial-a-prayer, and daily lunch-tray Scripture card provisions.[7] These and other entities contribute to antepartum patient empathy.

THE AUTHOR'S PERSONAL NOTE

My parents had eight children. I was number seven. They experienced five losses and never chose to provide details to me about those experiences. My purpose for writing this portion of the paper is to imagine the significance of parental connection throughout the complete life-span of an individual. My husband Roy and I experienced varying emotions at Jay and Justin's (our sons) graduations, weddings, the coming births of their children, etc. Connecting with new mothers is significant for me from my personal perspective. I present these two personal events I had with my parents to reflect the strength of parental connection that began when we were carrying our babies.

I was eighteen. The Bachelor Benedict Club in Norfolk celebrated the introduction of young ladies into society. All my six sisters had been likewise introduced when they were eighteen. All the girls wore white evening gowns, carried red roses, and wore arm length white gloves. We rehearsed curtsies and were told to inform our fathers that their role was to lend us a hand as we walked down the steps from the stage. My dad had three injured fingers that had been

---

6 Pet, music, and art therapy; support ministries sponsored by Baylor Hospital; Oncology and Cvetco Cancer Center. These services are provided to all patients and staff on the BUMC campus.

7 Daily public BUMC Telecare Dial-A-Prayer (214.820.2333); The Transplant and Digestive Services, service line from Baylor's OMM provides daily, Scripture/meal.

slightly severed in a printing accident during his youth. He asked me to place my gloved hand over his fingers to cover his hand as he escorted me off the stage.

As I recall this experience, I can only imagine the impact it had on my father. The event reflects for me the powerful ties children have with parents. I get emotional thinking about it because as humble as my father was at that moment, that sensitive moment provided a powerful connection that felt close, special, and memorable for us both. I imagine my sister siblings had similar experiences. And for all purposes, I can imagine his and my mother's thousands of memories were also paramount about major life events.

As the seventh child of eight children and the last one to get married, I recall another sentiment my mother had when each child left our home to get married. The plum tree in our yard was the place my mother stood under after the couples left for their new lives. My mother would moan and weep but seemed to reflect with godly expressions that the point of separation was not easy for her. She seemed to reflect a sense of accomplishment and love amidst her sadness. As an adult, I think she also appeared to hold in her heart deep prayers for what the couple would learn about the institution of marriage. My reflections were not as clear about my older siblings because I was in grade school.

This memory brings home the point that there is something intrinsically special about the bond mothers have with their children. I recall my mother's expression on our wedding photo with both mothers. She had the same look on her face I observed with my other siblings. She must have had both a sense of completion and awe as her nest was finally empty. I can only imagine the lifespans of all my siblings' births and major life experiences were echoed in her thoughts. Certainly, the birth processes were rehearsed. I find myself doing the same during important life events. For antepartum mothers this experience provides only the beginning of a lifetime of this pertinent initial bond between mothers and their babies.

I will now explore the wide range of cases, situations, and health-care conditions I encountered in the hospital. Later I will reflect on how my earlier teaching experiences in Virginia formed a huge connection to this project. All the patients were unique in this project and the chaplain residents and I wanted to learn more about the needs of these pre-term mothers. Our daily provisions were the result of a lot of hard work and constant prayer as you will observe in the preliminary classes. Let us now look at the needs of antepartum patients.

CHAPLAIN SUPPORT OF ANTEPARTUM PATIENTS

Wisdom in decision-making for antepartum mothers is advised as they experience agape love from themselves as well as their caregivers. When believing prenatal mothers agree to bedrest, they demonstrate their respect for God's word. Mothers can simply, "love one another (love their babies) as Christ has loved them [you] (John 15:12)." David Cook posits that the "kingdom life enjoyed in Christ comes when talents are properly used, enabling men and women to live a life in total obedience to the will of God."[8] Chaplains willingly provided empathetic support during these times.

Many felt needs of patients center on their babies alone. Many mothers who have medical conditions, center most of their thoughts on the growth of their babies. Mothers commit to doing whatever it takes to help improve their babies' conditions. The bedrest becomes an act of service for their babies. Some patients in the hospital cope by decorating their rooms, displaying their coming baby's names. Other mothers opt to leave the hospital "AMA" (Against Medical

8 David Cook, The Moral Maze: A Way of Exploring Christian Ethics (London: SPCK, 1983), 56. (Personal Entry by the writer--In much the same way, a pre-term mother's obedience to bedrest demonstrates her faithfulness in the process.)

Advice), due to babysitting, employment, financial, and other critical needs at home. Some of these mothers feel that they can spend
their time at home taking care of their coming babies and the other
demands at home. These antepartum mothers may get cabin fe-
ver and become anxious about remaining in bed for the prescribed
timeline. A few AMA patients readily return to the hospital. Patients
soon discover the stark reality that their own medical conditions and
the health of their babies are contingent on controlled hospital bedrest.

Lawrence Holst comments on pre-term mothers who address
their antepartum situations and commends those patients who
view their experiences as an "interruption." Holst observes: "I have
been impressed with the way many mothers handle (hospital experiences)—the women with incompetent cervics or spontaneous
rupture of membranes who are willing to devote months of time to
bedrest in hopes that labor will be delayed until their child's lungs
mature to the point of surviving birth. For others, the interruption
is experienced as hyperemesis (excessive vomiting, morning sickness) in early pregnancy, at times so severe that it causes a mother
to quit work earlier than planned."[9]

The antepartum mother needs a safe place to relay her feelings
while she is experiencing difficult medical conditions. Henri Nouwen
notes that Christian ministers can help (patients discover), "behind
. . . dirty symptoms, there is something great to be seen."[10] The pastor's lot is to listen to the problems expressed by the patient.[11] Christian leaders have the opportunity during visitations with patients to

---

9 Lawrence E. Holst, ed., Hospital Ministry: *The Role of the Chaplain Today*
(Eugene, OR: Wipf & Stock Publishers, 1985), 94-95.
10 Henri J. M. Nouwen, *The Wounded Healer: In Our Own Woundedness, We Can
Become a Source of Life for Others* (New York: Image Books Doubleday, 1990),
44.
11 Thomas C. Oden, *Pastoral Theology: Essentials of Ministry* (New York: Harper &
Row Publishers, 1972), 203.

"break through boundaries."[12] The pastoral provider seeks to "build bridges between Christ and the world,"[13] and to be able to "reach out for the hurt (in patients), an important mark of those who share Christ's ministry."[14] A minister then "becomes an agent of change," and the "voice of the Spirit" as compassionate care is provided to patients.[15]

Chaplains and others can provide a view of Christian hope and healing that helps patients dialogue about the beauty of the birthing process despite their medical prognoses. Psalm 139:13-16 reads, "you knit me in my mother's womb, and . . . for I am fearfully and wonderfully made..." deeply resonates with patients. A distinct wonder exists in the anatomy of a forming baby for antepartum mothers. Chaplains have the opportunity to assess the needs of a mother-to-be at her bedside. David Switzer, for example, asserts that pastoral care providers can initiate visits to believing patients by "determining whether the patient has a particular scripture in mind that is meaningful to them.[16] Neville Kirkwood suggests confrontational dialogue is not always the best practice. He states that "a pastoral visitor's own relationship with God through the Spirit will minimize the risk of rejection and maximize the possibility of fruitfulness because the timing will be right."[17]

LISTENING AND ATTENDING SKILLS

Chaplains and other spiritual supporters should choose to familiarize themselves with an entry-level knowledge of their patients' medical conditions. Chaplains must attentively listen to the needs

---

12 Nouwen, *Wounded Healer*, 41.
13 Oden, *Pastoral Theology*, 202.
14 Ibid., 203.
15 Nouwen, *Wounded Healer*, 43.
16 David K. Switzer, *Pastoral Care Emergencies, Creative Pastoral Care and Counseling Series* (Minneapolis: Fortress Press, 2000), 56.
17 Neville A. Kirkwood, *Pastoral Care in Hospitals* (Harrisburg, PA: Morehouse Publishing 1995), 130.

of the patient to determine wisely whether the patient welcomes medical dialogue. A couple of medical conversations, for example, seem to resonate with patients. Mothers-to-be often share sonograms with chaplains. Patients appear to maintain an element of hope during these times.

Sonograms are a source of tangible proof that their babies are maturing. Many mothers are connected to baby heart monitors at their bedsides. Their heartbeats are audibly heard. Nurses prefer that visitations are discouraged during these times. A medical motive in monitoring babies might determine why listening to the heartbeat of a baby is necessary. The well-being of the baby and the mother may be crucial for healthcare providers.

Chaplains may learn from other healthcare providers about several outstanding medical risks in the thriving of unborn babies with young gestational ages. Most mothers are aware of the pre-term medical risks in their prognoses but may prefer not to talk about them with a chaplain. Other mothers seem to prefer to discuss improvements alone. Patients often maintain a protective position of hope when they dialogue about their babies with a chaplain. Many mothers-to-be welcome dialogue and prayer. Patients dialogue openly about missing their children and families at home. They also openly discuss job challenges and agree to talk about the inconvenience of being in the hospital.

Trust developed over time can encourage dialogue between patients and chaplains. The chaplain does well to become familiar with medical terminology, but only to use the knowledge to support the patient's spirituality. Medical terminology is useful for chaplains at the floor multidisciplinary huddles. Some patients begin to realize in pastoral conversations that a team effort enhances the care of the whole person.

The following information is good reading about antepartum patients. The information is helpful because most healthcare providers agree that pre-term babies thrive at a better survival rate after delivery at no less than twenty-four weeks of gestation. Delivery is not recommended before that time. The following is a case in point. The information need not be quoted to patients by chaplains unless the dialogue is deemed helpful.

The age of a pre-term baby is determined by several factors. Specific ultrasound measurements of the unborn baby are determined from the "crown-rump" in early pregnancy (10.0/7 to 13.6/7 weeks of gestation) and/or the history of the woman's menstrual cycle. Accuracy in determining gestational age by early ultrasound is greater than or less than four days (twenty-five-to-twenty-six weeks). A much wider range is accepted (a minus six to a plus fourteen), as determined by the woman's last menstrual cycle. Sonograms, heartbeats, and other measurements and means become complicated as medical technology can determine potential health problems prior to birth.[18]

Chaplains might discover many levels of spiritual distress with mothers who have been placed on bedrest. On one of her pastoral care visits, I recall the recent weekly visitations to a mother carrying quintuplets. The pastoral care visits seemed beneficial during those quiet moments when the patient needed a listening ear. The antepartum mother's spouse's demanding job was in their hometown many miles away. Support from other family members and her church became paramount. A chaplain's visit serves as an additional avenue of spiritual support for the antepartum mother.

---

18 Thomas Berger, ed., "Perinatal Care at the Limit of Viability between 26 Completed Weeks of Gestation in Switzerland," *Swiss Medical Weekly* 10, no. 4414 (October 18, 2011): 2-3.

SOME RISKS PRE-TERM MOTHER'S FACE

Away from the hospital setting and before admittance to a hospital, mothers-to-be may find themselves lured to rising pharmaceutical options to acquire mood-smoothing, anti-anxiety, and anti-depressant drugs to help them with different levels of spiritual distress.[19] The role of a hospital chaplain and other spiritual helpers is unique. Chaplains seek to provide spiritual support to patients in the hospital, so they can cope with the duality of their medical conditions.

Antepartum mothers-to-be can build an ongoing basis of trust with healthcare providers when the present comprehensive information is presented with strong elements of support and sensitivity.[20] Antepartum pastoral support can assist patients as they deal with all things medical. Embryonic development research has shown that all 180 organs in the human embryo have significant functions in the human body.[21] These preterm organs need constant care by the antepartum mother and healthcare providers.

An entire body system is being developed in a coming childbirth. My own pregnancies and antepartum experiences of family and friends have guided me to invest more time and study to a woman's pre-natal needs. I also wanted to determine whether her spiritual health can affect a quality thriving of her baby. The health of the mother does affect her growing baby. When medical problems arise and the mother is placed on bedrest, one or more of the functions of the embryo might be affected. In looking at the clinical significance of patients' experiences, the following applies:

---

19 John Chafee, *Thinking Critically*, 8th ed. (Boston: Houghton Mifflin, Co., 2006), 435.
20 Berger, "Perinatal Care," 1-3.
21 Gary Parker, *Creation Facts of Life: How Religion and Spiritual Health Reveals the Hand of God* (Green Forest, AR: Master Books, 2006), 54.

In medicine, it would appear, words are not just words, and experiences in the venues of medical care are not just things that happen to patients. Words and experiences have a direct impact on patient's bodies; have the potential to influence illness for better or for worse. The experience of sickness, the experience of care, and the words of . . . caregivers are neither just kindness nor are they merely the necessary bearers of information that are peripheral with the main cause of the [medical condition]. Meaning . . . provides direct access to the sick or well person's body. It would seem worth learning about.[22]

Antepartum mothers are concerned about their own healthcare issues, especially if their conditions impact the health of their unborn babies. Mothers-to-be must often make crucial decisions about their unborn babies. The chaplain and other experienced members of the hospital perinatal/multidisciplinary team are needed to ensure quality care in the hospital.[23] Church and community-based visitations complement and do well to support the hospital staff. Medical information helps the staff measure vital information about the patient's condition. Some elements of spiritual distress may result from the physiological needs of both the antepartum mother and the survival of her unborn child. Spouses, other family members, and friends might also increase the feelings of spiritual distress in antepartum mothers.

Different behaviors in crisis management may often occur among couples during early pregnancy. For instance, a widespread divide may occur between the interests and expectations of antepartum couples, which may produce a linguistic battle of the sexes.[24] An antepartum hospital patient and her spouse might have to deal with lack of rest and an unspoken medical condition that they

---

22 Eric J. Cassell, *The Nature of Suffering and the Goals of Medicine,* 2nd ed. (Oxford, England: Oxford University Press, 2004), 242.
23 Berger, "Perinatal Care," 1.
24 Chafee, *Thinking Critically,* 266.

want to keep between them. Words of support and good listening and attending skills bring comfort and stability during times of spiritual discomfort.

ROLE OF THE HOSPITAL PASTORAL CARE PROVIDER

Important for a chaplain's awareness, is the mother's desire for pastors to ask good questions. . . opposed to giving solutions to their needs.[25] The history of the early church reveals ways chaplains can minister to patients in their spiritual distress. For this reason, some historical patterns and practices over time can serve chaplains. The Pastoral Rule by Gregory of Rome in 590 A.D. proclaims, the pastor (i.e., chaplain) must give attention to balancing the external function of . . . teaching and administrating the church (i.e. hospital) and its charitable work."[26]

The functions expressed here are essential in pastoral ministry to antepartum patients. Chaplains must exercise spiritual warmth and compassion as they meet the expressed theological needs of patients. Thomas Oden posits a definition of pastoral theology, defining it as a branch of Christian theology that centers on the office as well as the functions of the pastoral care provider.[27] Chaplains must work hard to advance their listening and attending skills with grace and divine sensitivity. Pastoral care providers do well to develop improved pastoral skill amidst the perceived needs of their patients.

Switzer contends that pastoral care is at its best when sensitive timing in dialogue allows for honesty and openness, which is a needed process in caring for others. Switzer also commends

---

25 Jill L. Snodgrass, "A Psycho-Spiritual Family Centered Theory of Care for Mothers in the NICU," *Journal of Pastoral Care and Counseling* (March/June 2012): 18.
26 Augustine Casiday, ed., Constantine to C. 600, *Cambridge History of Christianity*, vol. 2 (Cambridge: Cambridge University Press, 2007), 579.
27 Oden, *Pastoral Theology*, Introduction, x.

pastoral leaders to "trust the power of the Holy Spirit in human life; the process of caring is defined by attitude, relationship . . . with the use of concrete words in helpful facilitation to others."[28] Throughout the project, I addressed these and other pastoral skills needed to spiritually support antepartum patients.

I mention in this book some snippets from my doctoral paper, that might inform others about helpful ministerial practices we experienced with patients. We delved into theological themes that are introduced in Chapter 3, "Theological Reflections." Chaplains should desire to demonstrate the benefit of practicing a well-grounded faith to help patients in their *spiritual distress* (a definition).[29] Switzer notes that the pastoral care provider must reflect competence in the behaviors of helping with agape love.[30] Oden views pastoral

---

28 Switzer, *Pastoral Care Emergencies*, 11.
29 Sinclair Ferguson and David Wright, eds., New *Dictionary of Theology* (Downers Grove, IL: InterVarsity Press, 1988), 656-57; Nursing Care Plan, "Spiritual Distress," http://wps.prenhall.com/wps/media/ objects/3918/4012970/NursingTools/ ch41NCP_SpiritualDistress1055.pdf [accessed October 30, 2015]; and Lippincott Nursing Center (July 14, 2013), http://nursinginterventionsrationales.blogspot.com/ 2013/07/spiritual-distress. html-Minggu [accessed October 30, 2015]. Spiritual distress is defined here as a disruption in the life principle that pervades a person's entire being and that integrates and transcends one's biological . . . nature; Spiritual Distress, "Plans, Outcomes, and Interventions" (March 10, 2007), http://www.rncentral. com/nursing-library/careplans/sd-(NANDA) [accessed Oct. 25, 2015]; and T. H. Herdman and S. Kamitsuru, *Spiritual Distress 2015-2017: Definitions and Classification* (Boston: Wiley Blackwell, 2014). Herdman and Kamitsuru define spiritual distress as suffering related to the impaired ability to experience meaning in life through connections with self, others, the world, or a superior being. These definitions helped formulate the chaplains' working definition of spiritual distress in this paper. See also Harold G. Koenig, *Spirituality and Health Research: Methods, Measurement, Statistics, and Resources* (West Conshohocken, PA: Templeton Press, 2011), 54. Koenig is a physician, who completed his undergraduate work at Stanford University and received his medical training at the University of California in San Francisco, California. He serves as the Director of the Center for Spirituality, Theology, and Health at Duke University Medical Center, among other outstanding accomplishments in the field. The definition of spiritual distress in this paper is a disruption in the life principle that pervades a person's entire being that integrates and transcends one's biological . . . nature; a form of suffering related to the impaired ability to experience meaning in life through connections with self, others, the world, or a superior being.
30 Switzer, *Pastoral Care Emergencies*, 15.

leadership as service that is "properly defined as pastoral authority [for patients]," who "happily receive the good," as recipients of leadership that boldly guides [others] . . . based on what the flock yearns for and needs."[31]

Brian McLaren notes four points, among others, that might assist Christians in their care of others:

1. We must accept the co-existence of different faiths in our world willingly.
2. Having acknowledged and accepted the coexistence of other faiths, Christians should actually talk with people of other faiths, engaging in gentle and respectful dialogue.
3. We must assume that God is the unseen partner in our dialogue who has something to teach all participants, including us.
4. We must learn humility in order to engage in respectful dialogue.[32]

These talking points help chaplains utilize caution as compassionate care is provided to patients. A wide spectrum of people groups feel supported when chaplains allow patients to lead in the type of care they believe will spiritually support them in their hospitalization. The role of hospital chaplains moves patients from a place of spiritual distress to a place of spiritual connection. Healing begins to take place when patients reveal their spiritual hurts and bruises. I sought to identify some of those unpopular and sometimes unfamiliar theological places in the life of the antepartum patient. Other

---

31 Oden, *Pastoral Theology*, 53.
32 Brian D. McLaren, *A Generous Orthodoxy: Why I am a Missional, Evangelical, Post/Protestant, Liberal/Conservative, Mystical/Poetic, Biblical, Charismatic/ Contemplative, Fundamentalist/Calvinist, Anabaptist/Anglican, Methodist, Catholic, Green, Incarnational, Depressed-yet-Hopeful, Emergent, Unfinished Christian* (El Cajon, CA: Zondervan, 2004), 256-58.

themes were familiar and reflected the spiritual terms they might often hear in the local church.

The challenge for pastoral care providers is to utilize learned skills in helping the patients come to terms with what they are truly feeling as they carry their babies. The hope is that antepartum patients continue to leave the hospital with an improved level of spiritual support. My prayer for myself and others is to improve helping skills which leaves patients feeling fully supported. It is my desire that all would seek to provide improved care to patients. We must allow the Triune God to continue to minister to us about the spiritual needs of antepartum patients, at home, in churches, in community healthcare clinics, or other labor-and-delivery facilities. Additionally, my desire is to explore more helpful theological themes to assist pre-term mothers.

CHAPTER 2

Five Theological Themes

E ach once a week class session began with prayer and an expression of gratitude to the residents for agreeing to be a part of the project. We shared personal, vocational, and theological insights about the project to the chaplain residents.[33] All seven students who signed up for the project were present and the first class session went well. The five themes were introduced,

- God and Suffering
- Jesus, the Suffering Servant
- The Image of God
- The Church
- Eschatological Hope.

The presentation was in didactic form, welcoming dialogue with question-and-answer opportunities from the chaplain residents. I expressed gratitude to the chaplain residents for volunteering to be a part of the project. Clinical Pastoral Education Theological

---

33 The introductory session was led with a PowerPoint presentation and a description of the proposed weekly class overviews. Additionally, the actual PowerPoint presentation is in Appendix 2.

Education Certified Educator, Lauren Frazier-McGuin volunteered occasionally to sit in and participate in some of the class activities. Her participation appeared to equal (in essence) the level of chaplain residents. She was the class Certified Educator who volunteered her class time for this project, I found her silent support to be an asset.

I presented an overview of the six sessions, explaining in detail, the message intended in the five theological themes. In the explanation of the themes, I outlined my intentions to present theologians in the field who present biblical perspectives with the five theological themes addressed in this paper. Flyers with the themes would be presented to chaplain residents and the chaplain residents would present a more reader friendly version on the theological themes to the antepartum patients.

Each week, the plan was to distribute the flyers at the beginning of each class session. Chaplain residents were introduced to the two Spiritual Assessment Tools used for this study found in the daily Gateway/AllScripts and Eclipsys Electronic Documentation, and Focus Notations. Details of each class reflected hands on projects for all class participants. The class participants seemed eager to begin the process.

The next class scheduled class session was postponed for the following week because of a chaplain-wide lecture on human trafficking. The closing celebration was moved to May 23, 2018. The schedule for the day was followed carefully. The *PowerPoint* presentation ended, followed by a walking tour of the 7 Jonsson antepartum unit of the hospital, with an introduction to the 7J healthcare providers.

The formality in the introductions soon transitioned to cordial conversations among the staff and attending registered nurses. The healthcare staff and chaplain residents shared dialogue about their geographical states and locations that matched their selective counties and sometimes countries. The walking tour detailed a view of the 7J family/multi-purpose room/patient snack room, sonogram baby examination room, and general information about the nurses' station and charting area. The class returned to the original meeting room. After reflections and dialogue about the walking tour, I adjourned the meeting with prayer. The class was reminded to visit an antepartum patient of their choice during the week, remembering to chart their visits.

MEETING TWO

Everything in the session proceeded as planned. One student was unable to attend the session, and I later spent some one-on-one time with the student in a private session. The class accomplished most tasks as planned, which included a report about the patients they had visited over the weekend. In addition, the students had the unexpected pleasure of presenting stuffed animals provided by a *Baylor Foundation* donor. I reviewed the new theological theme, *Jesus, the Suffering Servant*.[34] The students distributed the encouragement flyers to the patients that I had personally chosen to ensure that chaplain visits would be welcomed. When the students appeared anxious about how to meet the spiritual needs of antepartum patients, I took time to discuss their concerns and allay their fears.

The class dialogued about Paul's writing in 2 Corinthians 1:3-7:

Praise be to the God and Father of our Lord Jesus Christ, the Father of compassion and the God of all comfort, Who comforts us in all our troubles, so that we can comfort those in any trouble with the comfort we ourselves receive from God, for just as we share abundantly in the sufferings of Christ, so also our comfort abounds through Christ. If we are distressed, it is for your comfort and salvation; if we

---

34 Chapter 3, "Theological Reflection."

are comforted, it is for your comfort, which produces in you patient endurance of the same sufferings we suffer. And our hope for you is firm, because we know that just as you share in our sufferings, so also you share in our comfort.[35]

The class dialogue led into a conversation about the role of a chaplain as it relates to antepartum patients. All agreed that the latter part of the Scripture referenced more mature Christians and may not be appropriate to quote with sick hospital patients (beginning with ". . . if we are comforted"). I facilitated a discussion about the theological positions and biblical referencing in this session. The theme of *God and Suffering* was distributed to chaplain residents for the patients who would be served by them on the following week. Chaplain residents distributed the same flyers to consenting antepartum patients on their next visitations during the week.

As the project director, I facilitated the chaplain resident's introduction of the flyers to patients and dialogued with them about ways to assess patients who welcome the dialogue on *God and Suffering*. Residents will read a poem, "The Children's Chaplain," with an activity and review, located in Appendix 5. The residents were encouraged to create a poem of their own, reflecting typical feelings of visiting patients on a night shift. The class also dialogued about intercessory prayer, the effects of Christian team ministry, and how God's glory is paired with his suffering. The class also dialogued about scriptures that reference Jesus the Suffering Servant, along with some "golden nuggets" from theologians on the subject. The scriptures that were highlighted referenced Matthew 25: 36b on being entrusted by God to serve, ". . . I was sick and you visited me," and Acts 4:27-30b, ". . . on the power of prayer and Jesus, God's holy servant."

---

35 *The Holy Bible: New International Version* (Grand Rapids: Zondervan Publishing House, 1984), 1579.

Chaplain residents sought to acquire biblical knowledge as they read Scripture and listened to applicable talking points about Jesus, the Suffering Servant. I spoke about the significance of Jesus and suffering as it relates to antepartum patients. Christ's humility, the suffering and glory of the servant is observed here (Phil 2:5-11). The God of the patriarchs raised up his servant as God's holy servant (Acts 3:26a and 4:27-30b). The project director led in a dialogue about a Reality/Wish List Room with chaplain residents. Chaplain residents planned to decorate a patient's room with a dream vacation/reality room for a single day.

The antepartum supervisor, the chaplains/learners, and project director dialogued about a possible production of a physical example of a fully decorated room reflecting a dream vacation. A drawing was held to implement the selection of the winning patient. The class assignment requested that chaplain residents verbally report Internet/faith-based searches at the next class meeting about antepartum patients and spiritual distress. These searches were voluntary and were presented in the next class session. Chaplain residents viewed a Baylor Spiritual Distress video.

MEETING THREE

The meeting began with the students' presentations of their Internet searches; one presented a psalm that she thought addressed spiritual distress and suffering. I showed the spiritual distress video and reviewed material from the previous week. Continuing the theme of suffering from the first two sessions, this week's theological theme was *God and Suffering*.[36] The students demonstrated excitement about their successful patient visitations. They gave detailed recollections of their patient visitations. The dialogues demonstrated their improved skill and increasing comfort in their ministry to antepartum patients.

36 Chapter 3, "Theological Reflections."

One of the chaplain's colleagues helped by managing my weekly online surveys.[37] The class completed the pre-test, a spiritual assessment tool; all participants completed these tests and on-line surveys until the close of the project. The chaplain residents continued to provide small pillow-like stuffed animals (pink and blue pastel) to patients they visited each week. A soft lullaby tune plays when an accordion type extension is pulled out from the stuffed animal. Chaplain residents noted that the patients were receptive to the stuffed animals.

The class again suggested a unique project to decorate a room with a makeshift dream vacation decoration for one antepartum patient. Students drew a name for the winning patient's room. The challenge for this approach was the increased turnover of patients who were discharging earlier than anticipated. Another factor was the gravity or critical nature of a mother's medical condition. The mandatory bedrest meant limited activity. The process would have to be repeated until a patient would be eligible for the dream vacation room make-over.

The class participants read the Children's Chaplain Poem and presented their own poetry at the next class meeting. Their poems reflected their hospital experiences. One chaplain resident detailed her own story that related to her own sister's prenatal hospital stay. Her poem reflected a difficult period in her sister's hospital experience. All the residents noted that the exercise in poetry was one of healing and meaningful reflection.

The class dialogued about the problems they might perceive in future dialogues with patients concerning evil and suffering. The project director and the class participants dialogued about the biblical references and the refreshing comments by Ashlock and Oden

---

37 Sherry Shanks is the Oncology Chaplain who assists OMM team members and clinical staff with crucial IT issues; also assisting with the same in this project.

referenced in Chapter 3, Theological Reflection.[38] God is at work and was at work as a means of salvation. Chaplain residents relished in the reminder that the Garden presented for humankind the need for relational wholeness. Discussion followed about the Fall and Theodicy that patients may ask of chaplains. Some dialogue occurred about the Imprecatory Psalms and the freedom believers have in dialogue about critical health conditions. I guided chaplain residents to visit another Antepartum patient during the week. I also facilitated the talking points to residents about *God and Suffering*. Residents received flyers on *God and Suffering*. Chaplain residents presented the same material to consenting patients.

I presented the theological theme of *God and Suffering* to chaplain residents that led into a discussion. I also introduced several quotations by theologians and preachers who have studied the subject of *God and Suffering*. I later led and facilitated a discussion about the theological positions and biblical referencing about the subject at hand. The theme of *God and Suffering* was distributed to chaplain residents. Chaplain residents distributed the same flyers to consenting antepartum patients on their next visitations during the week. I facilitated the chaplain residents' introduction of the flyers to patients and dialogued with them, ways to assess patients who welcome the dialogue on *God and Suffering*. Residents read the poem, "The Children's Chaplain," supported by an activity and a review, located in Appendix 5. The flyers for patients were graded down to simplify the subject in their delicate medical states. The students completed this activity and detailed that the poem resonated with them.

---

38 Chapter 3, "Theological Reflection," 35.

Meeting Four

I opened with prayer, with six residents present. *The Image of God* was the theological theme of the day.[39] The didactic was presented along with a welcoming dialogue with students. The student who did not report to class on the previous week read her poem relating to the Children's Chaplain learning activity. The student had written an insightful and touching poem and shared that the poem was composed on the anniversary of her sister's experience as an antenatal patient. Her account seemed to intrigue her fellow class participants to learn more about antepartum patients. The connection with their colleague seemed helpful in understanding the emotional state of antepartum patients.

The class reviewed the definition of spiritual distress before visiting patients on the antepartum floor. A chaplain resident reported that the patient she was to visit was unavailable, so the student left the encouragement flyer and other support material on her nightstand. The chaplain resident was later able to have a pleasant visit with the patient. The other residents' experiences with patients were phenomenal. They reported lengthy and successful visits. I was in awe of the students' enthusiasm. The residents reflected a significant mode of pastoral support to patients. The chaplain residents gave the impression that they emulated Jesus' image as they helped patients. Chaplain residents demonstrated Christ-like compassion and hospitality to patients based on their reported dialogues. The chaplain residents seemed to adequately adapt their ministry styles with godly compassion and human authenticity. The chaplain residents were instructed to read over the spiritual assessment tool regarding antepartum patients.

---

39 The questions from the spiritual distress instrument in Appendix 6 was used by chaplain residents and the project director to discuss the importance of the image of God in patients. The sentences and descriptions generate inquiries that focus more on the spirituality of antepartum mothers.

In conclusion, the discussion supported the statement that Christ's earthly ministry is an expression of his loving care. Jesus demonstrated this compassion in the lives of biblical characters such as the woman at the well, Peter, and the Emmaus disciple.[40] Chaplain residents gained knowledge about the *Image of God by* reviewing and listening to the didactic on the *Image of God*. I presented chaplain residents with encouragement flyers about *The Image of God*, followed by residents offering the same to patients. Props for role-playing were acquired from Baylor's supply chain from a clean linen room. After the class selected a patient for the virtual "Dream Vacation," I closed the session with prayer.

Meeting Five

I opened the class with prayer. The course was now well into week five, and the session went very well. After chaplain residents listened to a didactic about *The Church*, we dialogued about theological insights regarding the significance of the church found in the week's encouragement flyer. I dialogued about the spiritual journey genograms chaplain residents were challenged to complete. The genograms were to highlight the significance of individual, church, community, and family personalities in the lives of chaplain residents. The dialogue moved to the process need for the implementation of the genograms to antepartum mothers.

The class members completed their individual genograms, eagerly detailing the significance of helpful personalities in their lives. Many spoke of Sunday School teachers, school guidance counselors, high school coaches, and family members who had positive impact on their lives. The chaplain residents reported on how those days of early spiritual support would largely affect their pastoral ministries. I dialogued more about the new theme of the week, *The Church*. The genogram revealed the significance of the ministry of the church.

40 Kirkwood, *Pastoral Care in Hospitals*, 48-49.

The chaplain residents' positive connection with the genograms helped them transition the same assignment to antepartum mothers. The patients responded well to the spiritual journey genograms. Antepartum mothers relayed their positive memories of church youth groups, their pastors, caring babysitters, grandparents, as well as parents who helped them grow spiritually in life. Later the class went to the Baylor Cancer building/Cvetco Center to create paintings about one of the theological themes covered in class. My attempt to a pictoral Spiritual Journey genogram can be seen in the photographs particular to my story.

Some difficulty occurred in choosing a patient for the dream vacation project, as the 7 Jonsson patients were being discharged before the dream vacation project could begin. Most of the patients were discharged before this project could materialize. Other patients had prognoses that were of a nature that prohibited such activity for them. Some patients were too sick to be visited by non-medical staff per the physicians' and nurses' focus notes. The medical reports expressed in the 7J multidisciplinary huddles informed chaplains about patients whose medical conditions were critical. Because of patient turnover the class awarded the dream vacation winner tickets to a Jamaican restaurant. The patient delivered her baby who eventually went to the Neonatal Intensive Care Unit. The antepartum mother was the winner of the dream vacation. The mother was elated that we remembered her with her interest in having a "make-believe trip" to Jamaica. She thanked the chaplains for the dinner tickets.

The church functions as a welcoming agent for patients. A chaplain often represents the church (Gk. ekklēsia) or the patient's home community. Through pastoral support, antepartum patients can connect with their faith during times of spiritual distress. I introduced the significance of The Church as patients face their needs on the antepartum floor. Antepartum patients can address questions that help her name her feelings of spiritual distress from chaplain residents. Patients expressed the importance of the church and the role of faith in patient's lives. Shared hymn singing, hearing the songs of the church, and helpful scriptural passages have the potential to connect the patients with how much they miss worship activities.

The chaplain dialogued more with chaplain residents about the significance of evangelism to patients. With dependence on the Holy Spirit, receptivity with patients' interest in such a dialogue, might enhance a patient's spiritual health. However, chaplains were cautioned that verbal commitments to Christ must support the promotion of later home-church affiliation. We distributed the flyer and biblical theme on *Eschatological Hope*. I closed the class with prayer and well wishes for the coming week.

MEETING SIX

I opened the last class session with prayer and expressed my sincere gratitude to the chaplain residents for remaining committed to the project for the duration. The students completed their theological theme paintings, reflecting the five theological themes detailed in the encouragement flyers at the Baylor Hospital/Cvetco Center, located in the Sammons Oncology building. I shared a didactic on the topic of *Eschatological Hope*. The story unfolds with a mission field experience:

The story behind a small village boy's salvation came out of a story reported by Aggie (Aina) Hurst in a town where her parents had been missionaries in Africa. She was amazed when she learned that her mother Svea Flood who had died in childbirth had led a small African boy to Christ before she died. Aggie, now adopted in America, would learn that in that N'doleva village, he was now a leader (who was an expression of God's goodness and sovereignty) (Eph. 1:11,

"The plan of him who works out everything in conformity with the purpose of his will").[41]

This stirring event revealed a hope in ministry that had not been anticipated. The dialogue that followed between the chaplain residents and me, detailed the "seed planting," and the "watering," that chaplains provide to patients. The reality is that the life-changing events and their outcomes may never be seen in the lifetimes of the pastoral care providers.

I assigned patient visitations at random with no planned prerequisite visitations. I was elated to observe that the chaplain residents appeared eager to spend time with their patients. By this time, the students seemed to have lost their initial reservations about visiting unknown patients. The chaplain residents completed the on-line surveys and discussed their visitations in detail. The verbal reports given by the students demonstrated their growth and improved skill in providing care to antepartum patients. I plan to have certificates for each student at the closing celebration

I cautioned chaplain residents about offering false hope about specific medical conditions. The chaplain residents were at the same time encouraged to use the word hope in general terms. The patient may have their own view of hope and internally apply it to their faith base. I distributed the flyer on the biblical and theological theme on *Eschatological Hope*. During the week, chaplain residents presented the flyers to patients. I noted in the didactic that the church must be willing to admit our fallibility and sinfulness as we balance eschatological vision. Chaplain residents and the project director dialogued about hope and their coming babies. Hope was a theme that connected patients with their faith.

---

41 Randy Alcorn, *The Goodness of God: Assurance of Purpose in the Midst of Suffering* (Colorado Springs: Multnomah Books, 2010), 57. Alcorn's quotation is also written in Chapter 3, "Theological Reflection," 36.

Residents were next invited to create artwork in the form of mini-posters or small canvas paintings to present to the class, addressing one of the five theological themes. The Baylor Hospital/ Sammons Cancer Building/Cvetco Center is a place that invites creative projects by Baylor staff on a walk-in basis. The chaplain residents were asked to create artwork in the form of mini-posters or canvas paintings to present to the class on one of the five theological themes. Spiritual support and the patient's trust in a loving God must skillfully point to a God who is faithful and hears all the ardent prayers of all who call on Jesus, who is their ultimate hope. The center encourages artistic expression that may promote a form of art therapy.

Hope demonstrated to chaplain residents a theme that seemed intriguing to them. There were no hesitancies to broach the subject of hope because it was a familiar term for both chaplain residents and patients. Chaplain residents observed that eschatology for mothers meant holding on to Christian hope during their medical conditions. Mothers-to-be enjoyed talking about eternal hope and what they had learned from their pastors and churches. Chaplain residents seemed informed that in-spite of the more serious of medical conditions, patients and families seemed to hold on to hope. Some patients loved to sing the songs of the church that describe their hope in Christ. Hope may come in the form of acceptance of one's medical condition or other potential uncomfortable places for mothers. Antepartum mothers can also hold on to their faith in spite of their doctors' perceived prognoses of their coming babies. Chaplain residents were encouraged to ask patients about their coping skills. Residents were also asked to consider listening more rather than offering hope about patient's specific medical conditions. The discussions were fruitful in the chaplain's view.

Closing Celebration

As the project director, I welcomed the chaplain residents, to our closing celebration. In reflection, I was grateful for the Clinical Pastoral Education Theological Integration class and the Certified Educator, and the on-line survey facilitator in the physicians' dining room at BUMC. "Certificates of Completion" were awarded to each chaplain resident. The paintings of the five theological themes were displayed and explained by the chaplain residents to those assembled. The students reflected on the process and shared several testimonials about the personal healing they experienced as the five theological themes were addressed. The event took place on a day when staff chaplains and CPE faculty and managers were attending an off-campus conference in the city. I expressed my gratitude to all participants. The CPE chaplain residents, the Baylor IT Staff Chaplain, Sherry Shanks, and the Theological Integration Certified Educator, Lauren Frazier-McGuin, provided words of support as well. Discussion and much dialogue commemorated the closing celebration and the time together working on the goals of the project.

Plans to have a more inclusive closing did not materialize because of scheduling conflicts and the clinical need on the floors. The event took place on a Friday in the Physicians Dining Room. Doctors are not in large numbers on Fridays; which gave participants the welcomed surprise of meeting in the dining room in one of the physician's private meeting rooms. A group picture was taken to celebrate the success of the project. The physician's dining room was decorated in an exclusive restaurant style. The presentation and high-end food selections matched the celebration of the closing of the project. Again, the chaplain residents, the CPE certified educator, Lauren Frazier-McGuin, and the on-line survey monitor, Oncology Staff Chaplain Sherry Shanks attended the closing celebration. Project reflections, Certificates Completion Certificates, and displaying the residents' canvas theological theme paintings were the highlights of the event. I closed the celebration with prayer with heartfelt gratitude to all and their participation in the project.

CHAPLAIN RESIDENTS' BIOGRAPHICAL SKETCHES

The following biographical sketches detail the work of seven chaplain residents who volunteered to participate in this doctoral project. Aside from nurses and other healthcare providers who refer chaplain visits to patients, antepartum patients occasionally request regular chaplain visits. The group of chaplain residents in this project proved this suggested observation wrong. Patients requested repeated visits from chaplain residents to the point that some residents could not stop patients from wanting extended visits. In my opinion, theological integration class was a perfect forum for chaplain residents to learn the five theological themes they might consider presenting to antepartum patients. This is an introduction of seven residents who were willing participants to present a series of theological themes:

CZ is a single, thirty-five-year-old, female African American Clinical Pastoral Education chaplain resident. Born in Bay City, Michigan, she is the youngest of four children and has spent most of her life in Coppell, Texas. After graduating high school, she studied at the University of North Texas in Arlington, where she received her B.S. degree in criminal justice. She received her call to ministry in 2012 at the age of thirty and earned an M.A. degree in Biblical Counseling from Southwestern Baptist Theological Seminary (Fort Worth, Texas) in 2015. She is currently a second-year resident serving in Trauma ICU and Orthopedic floors. At the end of this residency, she will have nine units of Clinical Pastoral Education. Her post-residency goals are to continue her career in the chaplaincy ministry. CZ was always willing to visit the more challenging patients throughout this project. Many patients reported how much they felt spiritually supported by her. CZ posed questions to the group that generated good discussions and wrote a beautiful poem that was one of the many memorable assignments she completed.

LK is a commissioned and licensed minister of the Seventh-day Adventist Church. She completed a Master of Divinity degree and is working towards board certification as a Healthcare Chaplain. Before entering ministry, her career path included being a legal assistant, a risk manager in a healthcare setting, and extensive experience in the disability/healthcare insurance arena. She is a single white female who enjoys traveling, outdoor activities like hiking and golfing, and spending time with family and friends. At the onset of this project LK seemed somewhat timid about meeting the needs of patients with whom she was unfamiliar. By the end of the project she was focused and excited about meeting new patients suffering from a variety of healthcare challenges. She was conscious of budgetary needs as the project moved forward and was an eager participant in class assignments. She credited her family's support at an early age with regular Bible studies, both of which impact how she maintains her call to ministry.

KR is from Cedar Rapids, IA, where her parents and siblings still reside. She has experience in a variety of ministry settings, including international student ministry, young adult ministry, transitional living, and missionary service in Ethiopia. She was the former chaplain resident in Maternal Child Health in Women and Children's Services at Baylor, Dallas, and is currently pursuing a Th.M. degree at Dallas Theological Seminary. Throughout the project she provided compassionate care to patients and was known for her heartfelt prayers at their bedside. Her familiarity with antepartum patients proved helpful when 7J navigation issues arose, as her excellent connection with the antepartum patients for her peers was crucial in this project. Her administrative skills were superb as she balanced them with the broad and demanding needs of patients, staff, and her chaplain colleagues. I challenged her to broaden her scope amidst her orderly approach to service and to "trust the process" and rely on her faith when ministry challenges on the floors had unexpected outcomes. She accepted this challenge and experienced an amazing breakthrough with one of 7J's most challenging patients.

LPQ is from the Philippines and is an ordained minister in the Christian and Missionary Alliance. A clergyman with more than 2 decades of ministerial experience, he has pastored churches, participated in many leadership training venues, and had numerous teaching opportunities in many Asian countries. He earned a Bachelor of Theology degree in Pastoral Ministry, a Master of Divinity degree in Missions, and a Doctor of Theology degree in Systematic Theology. He is married with two children. LPQ was initially hesitant about the challenge of serving antepartum mothers and later developed pastoral compassion for them. LPQ overcame his reservations by exhibiting a notable level of compassionate care to spiritually distressed patients. LPQ boldly communicated each theological theme to the pre-term labor patients. LPQ posed many questions at the onset of the project for clarification. He showed much compassion as he detailed his visits with the patients during the group setting. This resident was attentive and very present when props were needed from another clinical area for role play needs of the group. He was acquainted with current trends and peer-reviewed articles that applied to the patient needs in this project.

EM, a Seventh Day Adventist, is a single Hispanic female from Veracruz, Mexico. Chaplain EM's parents, brother, and other family members currently reside in Mexico. After moving to the United States, EM earned a bachelor's degree in Theology and Biblical Languages and a Master of Divinity Degree. EM has participated in a variety of short-term mission trips in South America, Central America, and the Caribbean. She is passionate about proclaiming the Gospel message among many people groups; across different cultures. Even though she has not resided for a long period in the United States, she has quickly overcome many language barriers. As the current Maternal Child Health chaplain in Women and Children's Services her care of patients and their families is noteworthy. Her prayers and hopes for them have resulted in commendations by both patients and their families. EM has the unique and compassionate ability to calm their fears and to provide hope for patients who are experiencing despair and spiritual distress.

SC, an ordained Baptist minister in his twenty-first year of service, endorsed by the Baptist General Convention of Texas. He has been married for thirty years and has four grown children and three grandchildren. Following his retirement from the US Air Force as a Technical Sergeant, he earned a Master of Arts in Religion in Pastoral Counseling degree and a Master of Divinity degree in Pastoral Ministry. He and his family have ministered to churches in the USA in addition to serving as missionaries to Bulgaria and Germany. He was a notable leader throughout this project, always completing his assignments promptly and thoroughly, and was an outstanding team player among his chaplain resident peers. He provided a memorable Spiritual Journey Genogram that highlighted a remarkable, elderly female church member who was a strong and formidable Christian supporter to him that has lasted throughout his lifetime. SC's dry wit and humor kept the class lively and seemed to remind the group about memento items and encouragement flyers that were necessary during patient visitations. SC was the voice of reason when something unexpected was introduced in the daily activities of this project.

BR is a single Hispanic female who was an enthusiastic cheer-leader for this project from the first class session. Her support and full participation set the tone early on for a continued energetic class spirit that was contagious to all her peers. She has a Bachelor of Arts degree in Biblical Theology and has earned thirty-six hours towards her Master of Divinity degree. From San Antonio, Texas, where her family still resides, BR has an identical twin sister. She was a consistent team player within the project group. For her Internet search assignment, she boldly presented a scriptural passage that she found on-line. When the class went down to Baylor's Cvetco Center to complete their paintings on the five theological themes, she seemed excited and wanted to re-visit the center at a later class time to finish her project. I was pleased when she and another chaplain resident volunteered to visit with a patient who was a difficult case in the eyes of the 7J healthcare team.

CHAPTER 3

Theological Reflections

A s the antepartum woman is viewed through a broad theolog-ical lens, key pre-labor or antepartum biblical accounts are considered. Many biblical references might suggest a pre-term Christian women's embedded theology located throughout the biblical text. Instances detailed in the Old and New Testaments may present varied theological implications. One mother-to-be might ask, "What themes in the creation story, and in the Bible proper, might contribute to her embedded theology?" We begin this section on Theological Reflection with a tangible, spiritual, and theological approach to the dialogue and Christian theology that might assist patients as their spirituality is addressed.

BIBLICAL REFERENCES AND ANTEPARTUM WOMEN

A few pastoral hospital experiences I have observed over time reflect biblical and historical study. I recall some conversations with Christian mothers-to-be who dialogued about the biblical account and Eve's role in the creation story. Some Christian mothers hold several historical and biblical beliefs that are connected to their faith that have been gleaned from learned biblical teachings. The views are made known and remain embedded in their hospital experiences.

In Genesis, for instance, after the fall, Eve's contribution to the creation story is addressed. A few dialogues among women address the intimacy of the first man and the woman, which clarifies the "command and blessing of God," before the fall (Gen. 1:28)."[42] The Holman Bible dictionary describes this aspect of the creation story, "Humankind rests in the woman's capacity to bear children; the Creator's divine determination to preserve creation."[43]

The antepartum woman may also glean from other Old and New Testament biblical references that relate to the twenty-first-century Christian hospital patient. She may ask herself, "What is the significance of biblical accounts about pre-term and pre-labor patients, if any, that might inform her overall belief system?" Samuel's dedication account found in 1 Samuel 1-2:10, addresses barren Hannah's prayer as God answered her prayer for a son. Antepartum mothers review in this portion of the Bible, the power of prayer. The righteousness and sovereignty of God are celebrated in Hannah's song after the promise is fulfilled in the birth of Samuel.[44] Hannah, in this Old Testament scripture, was keenly aware of her barrenness. She took a leap of faith and prayed despite her medical state (her infertility).

Prayer and trust in God are crucial. The power and the spiritual importance of prayer are also observed in Isaac's prayer on behalf of his barren wife, Rebekah. This biblical account reveals Yahweh's

---

42 Trent C. Butler, gen. ed., *Holman Bible Dictionary: Exhaustive, Theological, Scriptural* (Nashville: Holman Bible Publishers, 1991), 472. This clarification is significant in the context that intimacy is not a sinful act and does not "suggest the knowledge of good and evil ... (as) sexual awareness."
43 Ibid., 472.
44 David S. Dockery, gen. ed., *Holman Bible Handbook* (Nashville: Holman Bible Publishers, 1992), 225.

answer to prayer over Rebekah's barrenness in Genesis 25: 19-23. In verse 23, "The Lord said to her, 'Two nations are in your womb, and two people within you will be separated; one people will be stronger than the other, and the older will serve the younger.'" Mothers-to-be can benefit from their prayer life with God as connection and dialogue with the Creator is crucial to the well-being of the mother.

In the Old Testament, we observe that Yahweh answered prayer in Exodus 1:15-20. The actions of the Hebrew midwives demonstrated their fear and homage to God. Pharaoh's instructions to the midwives Siphrah and Puah had been to slaughter all male Hebrew babies who were fast multiplying. This passage might suggest, indirectly, the essential nature of the medical profession as they work alongside pre-term women [and chaplains], as women face a variety of healthcare challenges.[45] Many believing doctors and nurses, other healthcare providers, as well as chaplains recognize Jesus as the Master Physician.

Christian antepartum women can know, "the true essence of the Gospel message," found in the New Testament as they come to grips with their medical conditions. The reality of the protection in the life of baby Jesus is evidenced through Joseph, his earthly father. Joseph's faith is depicted in his dream and "was directed to take his family to Egypt until it was safe to return to Nazareth."[46] Patients have the opportunity to overcome their fears about medical facts supported by their deep and abiding faith. This same Gospel message is supported by theologian Bultmann who posits that "Christians should accept the diagnosis and co-existence of inauthenticity (modern thinking, i.e., secular thinking) and the need for authentic thinking Christian choices. i.e., Christian thinking)."[47]

---

45 Berger, "Perinatal Care at the Limit of Viability," 1-3.
46 Butler, *Holman Bible Dictionary*, 815.
47 Cook, **Moral Maze**, 44-45. This portion of the paper supports the argument that Christian values and morality are important.

Christian prenatal women can better receive medical information when it is paired with their faith. The power of prayer allows for this dichotomy as believers are reminded to be of good cheer. In spite of the fact that they are in the world; Christ has overcome the world (John 16:33b). This discussion is crucial as some mothers-to-be cannot choose between the two perspectives. Therefore, in my opinion, pre-term mothers sometimes imagine that their medical problems exist because of their lack of faith or their practice in regular worship acts. The patient might determine that their imperfect lifestyles have resulted in some form of spiritual condemnation.

The New Testament offers stories that cause the antepartum mother to feel that she does not measure up to the standards of young Mary, the mother of Jesus. Mary's spiritual journey as the one chosen by God to give birth to the Messiah is a love and a God-story. As an African American woman chaplain, the dialogues about Mary in Luke's Gospel are significant. As the story unfolds, Mary faced ethnic, religious, and gender challenges. Mary's simplicity and instant submission to God were telling, as she faced the imminent birth of the Savior of the World. God's selection of Mary sends a unique message. Like Eve, Mary was chosen and equipped to do the work that God had called her to do. Likewise, the financial, governmental, ethnic, and religious challenges were real as she and Joseph faced the taxes of the land, the flight into Egypt and those who chose to destroy the Child. Luke describes Mary as a young woman of great faith, hailed in Mary's Song in Luke 1:46-56. It is interesting to note that Mary stayed with Elizabeth for three months. The essence of a caring and understanding relative is hailed here. Elizabeth was also carrying the child that Luke portrays as the prophet of the Most High, John the Baptist (Luke 1:76). Zechariah, John's father, also sang a song of celebration in Luke 1:5-25.

Then the prenatal woman might also focus on her maternal instincts and grapple with her on-going self-care, in comparison to the medical needs of her unborn child. She may ask herself a simple question about her mandatory bed rest, "Am I currently functioning as a good mother to my baby-to-be in the sight of God?" These inquiries are addressed throughout this portion of the project. I will detail personal perspectives, as well as some theological positions observed in patients, over time. The Wisdom Literature also affords patients the opportunity to address and utilize the Written Word in a unique way. Wise sayings from the Imprecatory Psalms, Proverbs, the flowery language of Ecclesiastes and the Song of Solomon seem to lift the spirits of long-term patients. The beauty and poetry expressed in the Wisdom Literature seem to be a source of healing for patients.

THE CHALLENGE OF PRESENTING A NEW LEADERSHIP MODEL TO NEW CHAPLAIN RESIDENTS

The theological themes in the lives of hospital chaplains are necessary to ensure quality pastoral care to antepartum patients. My work was to help chaplain residents reflect on the importance of improved skill in providing pastoral support. Jesus is the theological model; he demonstrated for all people the theology of acceptance, availability, accountability, care, sensitivity, obedience, witness, love, confrontation, renewal, and servanthood.[48] Robert Dale also presents biblical models for leadership found in both the Old Testament and the New Testament. Dale presents the leadership styles of "Nehemiah: The Catalyst (or Super) Leader, the Judges: Commander Leaders, Barnabas: Encourager Leader, and Saul: The Hermit Leader. The catalyst leader for Dale details that, "Nehemiah

---

48 Neville A. Kirkwood, *Pastoral Care in Hospitals* (Harrisburg, PA: Morehouse Publishing, 1995), 133. Kirkwood describes these theologies in detail in chapter 10, "Jesus—A Theological Model."

integrated his vision and concern for his people with a head full of goals and a heart full of empathy (67)."

Dale notes that "the commander leaders, were heroes, heroines, inspirational, charismatic, deemed interim rescuers and just 'got the job done (70).'" The encourager leader for Dale is applied to Barnabas who had the gift of developing friendships, vouched for others, and responded to the needy (72)." Dale concludes with the hermit leader. For Dale, Saul was initially a leader of great promise, but began to follow his followers, grew to be an unstable leader, lost his ability to influence or relate well to others (75).[49]

The residents in this project, in comparison, maintained growth in their care of patients, on the antepartum floor. The chaplain residents grew to be, as Dale describes, "encourager leaders," and improved their willingness to function beyond their comfort zones. This proved profitable for patients in my study. A chaplain's pastoral skill, in this way, is enhanced by working hard on the CPE helping skill competencies, the ardent study of God word, implementing strong life experience skills, and the theological themes among others introduced in this paper.

Maternal Child Health chaplains and chaplain residents do well to consider the pertinent theological themes prevalent in their own lives as it relates to their patients. Elisabeth Kurth notes, "A researcher's [chaplain's] own previous knowledge and beliefs function as a starting point to enter the 'hermeneutical circle' which describes the researcher's [chaplain's] circular movements between previous and

---

49 Robert D. Dale, *Pastoral Leadership: A Handbook of Resources for Effective Congregational Leadership* (Nashville: Abingdon Press, 1986), 66-77. Dale's book highlights biblical leadership models he names for the local church. The pastoral models help chaplains visualize styles that might help or hinder effective care and spiritual leadership to others At the time of this publication, Dale was a Professor of Pastoral Leadership and Church Ministry at Southeastern Baptist Seminary in Wake Forest North Carolina.

new understandings, as well as change between perspectives of a narrative as a whole..."[50]

A minister "looks for hope, on behalf of patients which 'prevents [ministers] from clinging to what [they] have and frees [them] from the safe place . . . [to enter that same place] with [others].'"[51] Antepartum women represent a unique patient population to new Clinical Pastoral Education (CPE) chaplain residents. CPE resident chaplains might experience some patients as "flat" or unwilling to talk about the many things that contribute to their mandatory stay at the hospital. As chaplain residents continue to work on their Association of Clinical Pastoral Education competencies, supported by seminary training, they might seek other helpful theological themes that may enhance their service to others.

The collaborative approach at Baylor asserts that many chaplain residents answer their pagers based on a quick request from the Pastoral Care page/triage operator. In a minute's notice, chaplain residents, in the course of a day may be called to serve patients in the Emergency Department, support families at a withdrawal of life support, attend to a palliative care/hospice patient or are called to settle down families in distress. Maternal Child Health antepartum patients' range of need is vast. Patient satisfaction is a major goal for the staff, and new chaplains may feel challenged about the many requests of antepartum patients. Most nurses refer these patients as they determine that many are lonely, in pain, or are worried about not being able to take care of their children at home. Many residents were successful in dialogue with patients. In this project, I chose to hand-pick patients, ensuring that the visits would be successful ones.

---

50 Elisabeth Kurth, "Crying Babies, Tired Mothers: Challenges of the Post-Natal Hospital Stay: An Interpretive Phenomenological Study," *Pregnancy and Childbirth* (2010): 1.
51 Nouwen, *Wounded Healer,* 45, 77.

Gene Wilkes' assertion in his book, *Jesus on Leadership*, also assists the chaplain residents in establishing a model of pastoral support for patients. The model directly applies to a model of servanthood that is vital in serving spiritually distressed patients. Wilkes' model impacts the well-being of patients as chaplains emulate Christ's love and compassion toward them. As observed in Wilkes' Principles, the necessary pastoral skill needed in providing care to patients is summed up in this way; "Humble your Heart, Be a Follower, and Take Risks."[52] Jesus humbled himself (Phil 2:8) enabling him to serve according to the will of God. Wilkes describes Jesus' story as having "A rags to riches beginning."[53] In-kind, the project director and chaplain residents have the opportunity to emulate Christ's model toward patients on the antepartum unit.

Toward the end of the project, no pre-selections were utilized in assigning chaplain residents to visit "safe" patients by the project director. Notable changes occurred as the chaplain resident's humility, welcoming spirit, and "meeting the patients at the table," positioned students to eagerly meet and greet patients before they had been introduced to their medical issues. The last two visits in week five and six were transformational as I witnessed a notable change in the chaplain residents. The chaplain residents seemed to race to the rooms, seeming confident about their desire to serve the patients with renewed spiritual confidence.

One can witness in the hospital, countless and "significant theological themes mentioned in the goals of this project.[54] My personal theology of spiritual care seemed to be reflected in like-minded care of patients by chaplain residents and was grounded in God's love for the world. After successful weekly visitations, tensions about caring

---

52 C. Gene Wilkes, *Jesus on Leadership: Timeless Wisdom on Servant Leadership* (Nashville: LifeWay, 1998), 25.
53 Ibid., 39.
54 Details for the Theological Basis for Ministry are in Chapter 4, "Critical Evaluation."

for these patients seemed to vanish. Chaplain residents were now both Christological and pastoral as they ministered to patients. They seemed to understand that the Father sent Jesus to demonstrate a level of compassionate care so that people who are alienated, sick, and in pain can also experience this love of God. The chaplain's role is to bring this love to prenatal mothers, their unborn babies, as well as their families. Nouwen asserts that [Christ's] "appearance in our midst has made it . . . clear that changing the human heart as well as our world is as interconnected as the two beams of the cross."[55]

According to Wilkes, Jesus' service to others was a "downward mobility, ending on the cross." It may also be understood as a way to "joy and peace that is not of this world." This writer's pastoral presence is likewise one of spiritual attendance toward others on the healthcare team, evidenced by human and divine compassion. This love is an ongoing message of hope demonstrated throughout the Bible. The residents seemed to capture this "servanthood" message with increased motivation."

When willing chaplain residents visited patients, this love of God helped patients feel that God cares and heals them—whoever they are and in whatever situation they find themselves. Several theological themes and spiritual needs arise in antepartum patients as they experience spiritual distress. Both chaplains and antepartum patients can observe Jesus' model of a Suffering Servant, who "leads others to trust him and to join him on his mission of reconciliation."

Some themes will be explored. In the book he edited, *Hospital Ministry: The Role of the Chaplain Today*, Lawrence Holst addresses the urgent call placed on chaplains to address faith and science through the window of theological knowledge. God's grace through justice and love contributes "to a moral ministry of sympathy, candor, and consolation."[56] Jesus' ministry led to the cross, which was

---

55 Goals are presented in Chapter 4, "Critical Evaluation."
56 Holst, *Hospital Ministry*, 12.

the ultimate sacrifice. His salvation work was driven by "love" and "obedience." The "universal language of salvation brings a message of hope for all."[57] Nouwen asserts that "faith is an attitude which grows from within."[58]

---

57 Wilkes, *Jesus on Leadership*, 242.
58 Nouwen, *Wounded Healer*, 30.

CHAPTER 4

Theological Themes Addressed in the Project

The theological themes covered in this project were:
1. *The Imago Dei, The Image of God*
2. *God and Suffering*
3. *Jesus, the Suffering Servant*
4. *Ekklesia, The Church or the Community*
5. *Eschatological Hope*[59]

These theological themes are supported by the definition of spiritual distress found in the Introduction of this project, Chapter 1.[60] Along with chaplain residents and antepartum mothers, I had the opportunity to explore the themes in the form of didactics, encouragement flyers, and dialogue. I led in teaching the themes to chaplain residents. The chaplain residents presented a more

---

59 These themes are detailed in the encouragement flyers seen in Appendix E.

60 Chapter 3, "Theological Reflections," 20.

reader-friendly version of the themes each week to patients in the form of tri-fold encouragement flyers. We all completed activities that reflected our understanding of the theological themes.

The first theological theme focuses on the *Imago Dei, The Image of God*, a topic that embraces humankind's identity in Christ. In Stephan Seamand's book, *Ministry in the Image of God*, he challenges the reader to never "give up" and to "fully surrender" to "Christ's lordship."[61] Antepartum patients need to hear this "good news" from Christian [pastors], that "behind the dirty curtain of their 'painful symptoms . . . [they see] the face of Him in whose image we are shaped."[62] According to Garrett, the task of Christian theology is... practical. Christian theology helps move human beings into a redemptive fellowship with God and growth in "God-likeness."[63] Antepartum women can also benefit from Nouwen's assertion that the minister "tries to help [patients] recognize the work of God in themselves," to help [patients] "those who are searching."[64]

The image of Christ is that to which humankind is to be conformed. The Image of God is detailed many places in the biblical text: Rom. 8:29, "For those God foreknew he also predestined to be conformed to the likeness of his Son . . ."; 1 Cor. 15: 49, "And just as we have borne the likeness of the earthly man, so shall we bear the likeness of the man from heaven"; 2 Cor. 3:18, "And we, who with unveiled faces all reflect the Lord's glory, are being transformed into his likeness with ever-increasing glory, which comes from the Lord, who is the Spirit"; and 2 Cor. 4:4, "The god of this age has blinded the minds of unbelievers, so they cannot see the light of the Gospel of the glory of Christ, who is the image of God."[65] Chaplains can

61 Ibid.; and Seamands, *Glad Surrender*, ch. 4, 87.
62 Nouwen, *Wounded Healer*, 44.
63 James Leo Garrett Jr., *Systematic Theology: Biblical, Historical and Evangelical*, vol.1, 4ᵗʰed. (Oregon: WIPF & Stock, 1990), 7.
64 Nouwen, *Wounded Healer*, 49.
65 James Leo Garrett Jr., *Systematic Theology: Biblical, Historical and Evangelical*, vol. 1, 4th ed. (Eugene, OR: WIPF & Stock, 1990), 7.

present to patients the image of Christ perspective; "Christ within each one of his children is indeed the Hope of glory."[66] Holst introduces a theology of parenthood "to a God-centered partnership as co-creators."[67]

Neville Kirkwood explains that "patients need to see the Christ image and touch reflected in chaplains at the bedside. Neville addresses Jesus' sensitive handling, bringing comfort and peace to the woman at the well, the widow of Nain, Mary of Magdalene, Mary and Martha, his tormentors at Calvary, and Peter and the Emmaus disciples."[68] Henri Nouwen concludes that "the imitation of Christ means to "live... life as authentically as Christ lived his."[69] "Ministers must always be agents of prayer, ones who are able to recognize in others the face of the Messiah and make visible that which is hidden, make touchable what was unreachable."[70] Seamands also posits the "ministry is participating with Christ in his ongoing ministry as he offers himself to others through us."

Many antepartum patients may experience a range of emotions reflected in feelings of "isolation, lack of control, confusion,"[71] and "anger,"[72] about their medical situations in their pre-delivery experiences. Nouwen posits that many "have become unfamiliar with and even somewhat afraid of [considering], the deep movements

66 Stephens Seamands, *Ministry in the Image of God: The Trinitarian Shape of Christian Service* (Downers Grove, IL: IVP Books, 2005), 145.
67 Holst, *Hospital Ministry*, 80.
68 Kirkwood, *Pastoral Care in Hospitals*, 48-49.
69 Nouwen, *Wounded Healer*, 99.
70 Kirkwood, *Pastoral Care in Hospitals*, 47.
71 Ibid.; and Snodgrass, "Psycho-Spiritual Family-Centered Theory," 18, fn. 11.
72 Andrew Lester, *The Angry Christian: A Theology of Care and Counseling* (Louisville, KY: Westminster/John Knox Press, 2003), 13. Anger is a near-universal response from antepartum women and their families; rather than push them further away from God, anger can be an avenue through which one expresses her need of God (see the imprecatory Psalms). One view of imprecation supports the belief that God's "covenant love" intervenes in the lives of believers (Ps. 5:7 [mercy . . . and reverence . . .]; 59:10   [. . . my loving God], and 16-17 [my Strength . . . my fortress, my loving God]). Butler, *Holman Bible Dictionary*, 692.

of the Spirit, in the midst of their despair."[73] One might ask how, for instance, being formed in the image of God can help antepartum patients address anger. For Andrew Lester, anger is found to be the least understood of the emotions in patients and families. Suggesting a unique and theological approach to this emotion, he says that "anger has its origin in creation," a "basic ingredient, connected to the embodiment of the *Imago Dei*, a true gift from God."[74] Lester's position provides a model for all other feelings patients may experience on the antepartum floor. Nouwen supports a similar position on the significance of Christlikeness as believers relate to others.[75] In Nouwen's view, compassion and hospitality help the minister connect and help patients in their despair. Personal healthcare challenges are best experienced when observed through the lens of a loving Savior.[76]

A second theological theme for antepartum mothers is *God and Suffering*. Evidenced in Larry Ashlock's writing, humankind can be comforted in the knowledge of "the final triumph in his [Christ's] life of good overcoming evil." Through Paul (God's) divine providence is evidenced in Romans 8:28 (...in all things God works for the good of those who love him...).[77] In the theological reflection of his work, Ashlock presents to readers the reality that God is "not destructive, but eternally redemptive; the author of all that is good."

Additionally, Ashlock addresses the problem of evil and suffering in the Fall and in the Creation Story. Amidst the cosmic chaos,

---

73 Nouwen, *Wounded Healer,* 38
74 Lester, *Angry Christian*, 13.
75 Nouwen, *Wounded Healer*, 40-41. Nouwen states that "compassion must become the core" of how we relate to others; the compassion of God with man [is made] visible in Jesus Christ, credible in his own world.
76 As a breast Cancer survivor, this statement is a personal reflection about the agape -love needed throughout challenging healthcare conditions.
77 Larry Ashlock, "Equipping Christians to Deal Effectively with the Problem of Evil and Suffering" (D.Min. proj., Southwestern Baptist Theological Seminary, 1985).

God was at work to provide "a means of salvation." The root of human suffering began with Original Sin in the Garden.

One common question individuals (especially antepartum mothers) might ask is, "Why did this happen to me?" Readers observe in Ashlock, the broad address to the moral evils evidenced in humankind.[78] For antepartum patients, many might find meaning to Seamands' position that humankind has a strong need for "relational wholeness." Seamands also notes as does Ashlock (concerning Adam and Eve, in reference to the Fall), that "as a result of their sin, all of their relationships, with God, each other, and the natural world were radically affected."[79] Seamands also offers that, "living in the fallen world we inherited from them means living in a world with broken relationships.[80] For the antepartum mother, this theme may apply to a good number of their familial and relational needs.

One who is experiencing spiritual distress may experience right thinking and right movements toward all that is holy. Nouwen presents the perspective that "pain" in the minister's life can "convert weakness into strength" and can be offered as a "source of healing to those who are often lost in the darkness of their own misunderstood sufferings."[81] In the chapter entitled, "Wanting More Clarity and Wrestling with the Reason for Our Suffering," Randy Alcorn expresses in his book that an individual's great tragedy, once experienced, produces an indelible print in the person's memory (the selfless comment): "I have thought, if this thing was going to happen to someone, it was better to happen to me, with my faith in God."[82] I recall a testimonial from a Christian patient who was suffering from the same condition her mother had before childbirth. Alcorn's

78 Ibid. 4, 7, 11, and 13.
79 Ibid.
80 Scott Witsen, "What Do I Fear When I Fear My God? A Theological Reexamination of a Biblical Theme," *Journal of Theological Interpretation* 9, no. 1 (2015):
81 Nouwen, *Wounded Healer*, 87.
82 Ibid.; and Alcorn, *Goodness of God*, 101.

assessment holds true in this case. The antepartum patient noted that she would rather bear this burden than have one of her younger siblings experience her condition.

As presented before, I reiterated this theme and presented more theological and biblical referencing on the theme, *God and Suffering*. The theme flyer on *God and Suffering* was distributed to chaplain residents. Chaplain residents passed out the same flyers to consenting antepartum patients on their next visitations during the week. I facilitated the chaplain resident's introduction of the flyers to patients by rehearsing the theological themes in the encouragement flyers. I dialogued with chaplain residents about ways to assess patients who welcome dialogue about *God and Suffering*.

Thomas Oden addresses suffering in his challenge to pastors to "learn to speak wisely," as they witness great misfortune over the evil and suffering experienced by people under their care. Oden rightly suggests that pastoral care providers "cannot say nothing." The reality is that the Bible offers no fixed answers for pastors as they minister to patients who cannot understand their suffering. Pastors can continue to seek to console patients, says Oden, ever focusing on [God's] goodness and power amidst the suffering.[83] Lawrence Holst reminds chaplains of Jesus' words in the Sermon on the Mount: "Blessed are the meek, for they shall inherit the earth" (Matt. 5:5, ESV). Holst maintains that "in brokenness one finds wholeness; in self-surrender, self-discovery; in death, and in life."[84] Since chaplains can help patients in their suffering, Holst provides a perspective on how they might help women during stressful times of need. Holst further presents a ministerial approach to help patients in their illnesses and their need for healing of the human spirit. He concludes that "hospital ministry is a crisis ministry, where a person's needs are identified in spiritual language—hope, trust, love,

83 Oden, *Pastoral Theology*, 226.
84 Holst, *Hospital Ministry*, 197.

and acceptance."[85] Herdman and Kamitsuru also define spiritual distress as suffering related to the impaired ability to experience meaning in life through connections with self, others, the world, or a superior being.[86]

As outlined by Neville Kirkwood, suffering addresses "a theology of renewal." In his ministry, Jesus himself experienced power drawn from him in every miracle; throughout his ministry he was aware of "the spiritual, emotional, and physical experience," unto all to whom he ministered. Preterm mothers can also find a quiet place of respite, just as Jesus sought and experienced planned "refuge and retreat."[87] Antepartum women have the opportunity to observe biblically-based truths about suffering. Thomas Oden asserts that "God suffers with us," found in Heb. 2:9 (now crowned with glory and honor because he suffered death . . .) and believers are not alone in their suffering. There is an eternal victory in God, and Jesus is our model for hope. Ministers are "constantly invited to help others overcome" their fears by "entering into it with them, and to find in the fellowship of suffering the way to freedom."[88] It is only when pastors enter into communion with others' "human suffering . . . that relief can be found."[89]

The third theme addresses Jesus, the *Suffering Servant*. In his sermon in the Acts of the Apostles, Peter states that the God of the patriarchs was said to have "raised up his servant" (v. 3:26a). In the prayer at Jerusalem, Jesus is referred to as "God's holy servant" (4:27-30b). Christ's humility is observed in Philippians 2:5-11 and in Isaiah 52:13-53:12. Christ's "self-emptying" ends at the cross where the suffering and the glory of the Servant are observed. Christ

---

85 Ibid. 85.
86 Herdman and Kamitsuru, *Spiritual Distress* 2015-2017 (also found in fn. 30).
87 Kirkwood, *Pastoral Care in Hospitals*, 131.
88 Nouwen, **Wounded Healer**, 77.
89 Ibid.

denied himself for the sake of others; believers are called to walk the same road, emulating the attitude that Christ had [at Calvary]; here, God's glory is paired with his suffering.[90]

As individual mothers respond to what God has done in Jesus, this helps them in their relationships with God.[91] Garrett suggests another Greek term, *pais theou*, meaning "Servant of God." This term is used both in pre-Christian Judaism and in the New Testament with two meanings: "Child of God" and "Servant of God."[92] Patients who are believers can share His sufferings, thus sharing His eschatological glory.[93] Nouwen posits that in his story and in his servanthood, Jesus "presents... a new fullness by making his own broken body the way to health."[94] The theological significance of the "promised King" is also proclaimed as the Servant King in the Gospel of Matthew. Hospital chaplains can serve antepartum patients through empathetic listening, intercessory prayer, and team ministry.[95]

In 2 Corinthians 7:1, the Apostle Paul further reminds the community of faith to "...purify themselves from everything that contaminates body and spirit, perfecting holiness out of reverence for God." Chaplains can comfort those who suffer from the biblical mandates Matthew addresses in Matthew 25:36b, "...I was sick and you visited me." Additionally, the apostle Paul addresses suffering in 2 Corinthians 1:3-7:

> Praise be to the God and Father of our Lord Jesus Christ, the Father of compassion and the God of all comfort, Who comforts us in all our troubles, so that we can comfort those in any trouble with the comfort we ourselves receive from God, for just as we share

90 John N. Oswalt, ed., *From Biblical Text . . . To Contemporary Life*, Isaiah, NIV Commentary (Grand Rapids: Zondervan, 2003), 588.
91 Ibid., 143.
92 Garrett, *Systematic Theology*, 8.
93 Ferguson and Wright, *New Dictionary of Theology*, 668.
94 Nouwen, *Wounded Healer*, 82.
95 Dockery, *Holman Bible Handbook*, 567.

abundantly in the sufferings of Christ, so also our comfort abounds through Christ. If we are distressed, it is for your comfort and salvation; if we are comforted, it is for your comfort, which produces in you patient endurance of the same sufferings we suffer. And our hope for you is firm, because we know that just as you share in our sufferings, so also you share in our comfort.[96]

Another significant theological theme needed for antepartum mothers is one that represents the *ekklesia*,[97] *church*, or the *community* that may not exist during their stay at the hospital. Through pastoral support, antepartum patients can connect with their faith during times of spiritual distress. A loving community of faith constitutes *The Church* or a fellowship of believers who work together for the well-being of one another's spiritual health.[98]

Antepartum patients can address questions that help name their feelings of spiritual distress in the absence of their ongoing faith traditions. Pastors have the potential to become "Good Samaritans" when their work and support of others bridges the gap between church and the needs that are vast in patients' home communities.[99] For Nouwen, it is the welcoming "hospitality" of the minister that evolves into "community as it creates a unity based on the shared confession of our basic brokenness and on a shared hope."[100] The hospital chaplain may represent the church for patients. To paraphrase theologian Rick Warren, who states, "The church must offer people something they cannot get anywhere else."[101] This statement

96 *New International Version* (Grand Rapids: Zondervan Publishing House, 1984), 1579.
97 The church has played a significant role in the life experience of my spiritual development as a chaplain.
98 Mark Driscoll and Gerry Breshears, Vintage Church: *Timeless Truths and Timely Methods* (Wheaton, IL: Crossway Books, 2008), 40.
99 Seward Hiltner, *Theological Dynamics* (Nashville: Abingdon Press, 1972), 123-24.
100 Nouwen, *Wounded Healer*, 93.
101 Rick Warren, *The Purpose Driven Church: Growth Without Compromising Your Message and Mission* (Grand Rapids: Zondervan Publishing House, 1995), 48.

can be supported by the ministry of a chaplain as pastoral care providers emulate the work of the church.

When appropriate, a chaplain might consider addressing the following: Elizabeth J. Taylor asks healthcare providers the question in the title of her book, *Spiritual Care: Evangelism at the Bedside?* The question asked is if evangelism at the bedside is acceptable. Taylor offers the significance of adequate care: "by listening deeply providers allow the patient to give voice to her inner experience." Taylor notes that the spiritual distress of the patient may bring potential hope when the distress is engaged. "It is acceptable to offer spiritual support as part of care when a patient asks for it," she adds. Additionally, Taylor suggests that healthcare providers should respond to patients with brief restatements, open-ended questions, or reflections of feelings to allow for explorations of one's own spirituality.[102]

David Switzer provides a well-thought-out process for patients who do not seem open to receiving support from available spiritual resources. If patients are unreceptive to his suggestions, he encourages dialogue and follow-up visitations that are not to be rushed. Switzer positions himself to offer patients help to assist them in following-through with his suggestions.[103] Switzer details the need for pastors to emulate agape love to patients and their families in distress, even when social justice and past church experiences have shadowed their view of the world.[104]

The fifth and final theological theme in this project has the potential to center patients on the *Eschatological Hope* they have in the coming age of Christ's appearing. Nouwen states that "hope makes it possible to look beyond the fulfillment of urgent wishes and pressing desires and offers a vision beyond human suffering and even

---

102 Elizabeth Johnston Taylor, "Spiritual Care: Evangelism at the Bedside?," *Journal of Christian Nursing* 28, no. 4 (2011): 194.
103 Switzer, *Pastoral Care Emergencies*, 186.
104 Ibid., 17.

death.[105] The following story of an antepartum mother addresses a hope that would manifest itself in the lives of others long after that event (this reference will also be in a later quotation in this book).

> The story behind a small village boy's salvation came out of a story reported by Aggie (Aina) Hurst in a town where her parents had been missionaries in Africa. She was amazed when she learned that her mother Svea Flood who had died in childbirth had led a small African boy to Christ before she died. Aggie, now adopted in America, would learn that in that N'doleva village, the young boy who was saved was now a leader (an example of God's goodness and sovereignty). (Eph. 1:11, "The plan of him who works out everything in conformity with the purpose of his will").[106]

Comforted by his hope in Yahweh, Job proclaimed a hope that did not falter despite his situation (Job 12:13 "To God belong wisdom and power; counsel and understanding are his"), as expressed by editors Easley and Morgan. Christ's lordship in the church helps in the dialogue that the issues of this life are a foretaste of the feast, a preview of the new heaven and new earth.[107] For instance, a mother may have to cope with carrying twins to term with the awareness that one of the twins will not thrive at all. The chaplain might present to the prenatal mother an eschatological perspective about the underdeveloped twin. The twin who will not be born alive may have a powerful impact and eternal purpose in Christ's kingdom to come.

Gary Habermas notes that those who express a need for worship during times of despair can think about God alone, pointing only to him (Matt. 4:10). Those experiencing spiritual distress can express their gratitude for divine presence (Eph. 5:20 "always giving

---

105 Nouwen, *Wounded Healer,* 76.
106 Alcorn, *Goodness of God,* 57.
107 Kendall H. Easley and Christopher Morgan, eds., *The Community of Jesus: A Theology of the Church* (Nashville: Broadman and Holman Publishers Group, 2013), 258.

thanks to God the Father for everything, in the name of our Lord Jesus Christ."), and praise God despite their circumstances (Heb. 13:15 ". . . let us continually offer to God a sacrifice of praise—the fruit of the lips that confess his name.").[108] Nouwen further details that ministers express hope to patients that "offers a vision beyond human suffering [built] on a promise given to him."[109]

On the theme of *Eschatological Hope*, theologian Richard Hays states in the conclusion of his book that the church must be a "community living in the conformity to the paradigm of the cross... standing as a sign of the new creation promised by God." Hay's warning to the church is to never forget the "eschatological reservation," the "not yet," which is crucial to understanding the "new creation."[110] Hays's position on hope can help antepartum mothers focus adequately on the spiritual hope they have in Christ Jesus' appearing. Hays states that the church must be willing to admit, "Our own fallibility and sinfulness," as believers balance "eschatological vision" and the present. "In the midst of a creation that still groans, awaiting redemption," Hays suggests that the church (i.e., antepartum patients through guided dialogue with chaplains) must continue to "hope, pray, and work: more closely conformed to the will of God, as disclosed in Scripture."[111]

ARE THE THEOLOGICAL THEMES IN THIS BOOK ADEQUATE FOR SUPPORTING HOSPITAL PREGNANT MOTHERS?

---

108 Ibid.; and Gary R. Habermas, *Why is God Ignoring Me? What to Do When It Feels Like He's Giving You the Silent Treatment* (Carol Stream, IL: Tyndale House Publishers, 2010), 102-3.
109 Nouwen, *Wounded Healer*, 76.
110 Richard Hays, *The Moral Vision of the New Testament: A Contemporary Introduction to New Testament Ethics* (New York: HarperCollins Publishers, 1996), 469.
111 Ibid. 470.

Looking at specific theological themes was significant and informative throughout the project. *Hope* was the theme that most resonated with patients when chaplains provided care. The word alone meant so many things to many mothers-to-be. When prognoses seemed grave, at the moment, mothers seemed to want to hold on to *Hope* whether she understood the prognosis for herself or for her baby. Suffering was the least popular subject; however, many ante-natal mothers commented on the biblical aspects of suffering outlined in the Bible. Most mothers-to-be provided affirming comments about the flyers that addressed *Jesus the Suffering Servant* and *God and Suffering*. The subject also resonated with chaplain residents who seemed reluctant to present the flyers with the word *Suffering* on them.

I was intentional in my use of words and phrases in the flyers. Most discussions with chaplains and patients took place after visitation, and after they read the flyers. The patient seemed informed about Adam and Eve and the "Fall." All the information that was included in the Theological Reflection segments of this paper was paraphrased for the flyers. Patients seemed more familiar with *The Church* and relished being made in the *Image of God*. The patients began to expect the flyers each week, along with plans to address other themes in the future. A description of how I experienced antepartum mothers follows:

Hospital antepartum patients may spend many nights in the hospital upon the advice of their physicians. A mother with a pre-term pregnancy might have many reactions to this advice, with responses ranging from welcoming the much-needed bed rest to frustrations about leaving their children and families over long periods of time. This study came as a result of those memorable moments I experienced visiting antepartum patients. The visits were usually good ones.

The element of the unknown appears to be the unspoken reality in this chaplains' conversations with mothers-to-be. Patients appear open to talking about how they feel physically, emotionally, and spiritually. Pre-term mothers also seem excited when mentioning the names of their coming babies or participating in upbeat conversations. Could there be another spiritual dimension that the chaplains are not addressing? The intention of this study was to grasp a renewed perspective about spiritual distress in antepartum patients. Are these mothers, in fact, experiencing vast levels of spiritual difficulty, and if so, what pastoral approaches are needed to assist them amid severe medical conditions?

Many questions were addressed in this paper—could there be additional ways to identify spiritual distress in antepartum patients at Baylor Medical Center in Dallas, Texas? Are there other claims that might support or deny the need for added spiritual awareness that chaplains might discover and address with prenatal mothers?[112] What significant themes in this project inform the masses about antepartum women? Might a more intensive study about teens and unwed mothers serve their concern more directly? Could there be some meaningful correlations between antepartum and postpartum spiritualities among women?

The experience was a rich one for me. The opportunity to work with the BUMC chaplain residents was memorable. Pastoral leadership to chaplain residents who came from a plethora of faith traditions, cultures, and theological perspectives was both refreshing and challenging. In reflection, the results of the surveys could have included more theological themes that encompass the antepartum world of mothers at BUMC. The establishment of a formal and universal definition of spiritual distress may help those in the future who study this service line in the hospital.

---

112 The prospectus abstract, vi.

The project helped the participants reflect on and identify their personal theological perspectives. The unique population of women in the antepartum world presented an opportunity for the participants to explore the complex needs of mothers carrying babies. The distress factor was even more complex as the mother's distress might have been relational to her coming babies "medical distress." The medical distress of the baby may influence how the mother copes with her spirituality before delivery.

Therefore, I conclude that this exhaustive study has heightened my own theological perspectives about the prenatal mother. My personal and family history is informed by the research presented in the original project that grew into a more local and global endeavor. I also recall recent conversations with helpful doctors and other healthcare providers who expressed their Christian faith as they dealt with challenging medical conditions. I also learned new theological perspectives from my chaplain colleagues, theologians, physicians, other researchers, and healthcare providers.

I learned first-hand the necessity of hard work by chaplains and other medical professionals whose faith and theology might be difficult to measure (in their care of antepartum mothers), through formal healthcare instruments alone. If there is such a measuring tool out there, I hope the results will assist other chaplains in figuring out how or whether these patients' levels of spiritual distress could be measured with a proper, viable and formidable tool. It is my opinion that this study accomplished more than anticipated. The test results could not measure the support antepartum patients experienced from chaplains and many other avenues of support. Only the Creator God; Jesus, the Christ; in the comforting power of the Holy Spirit can reflect an accurate picture of the meaningful care chaplains and others on the healthcare team provided antepartum patients in this project and then the resulting publication.

IDEAS FOR CONTEMPORARY MINISTRY

The pre-labor woman in the twenty-first-century hospital is unique, as she faces various forms of spiritual distress explored in this paper. The results of this study might help broaden the ministerial awareness of chaplains, ministers, church pastors, counselors, and related healthcare support initiatives. The findings of this study may serve as a resource to address spiritual distress at varying levels, with the spiritual well-being of antepartum mothers as the primary objective. The research in this paper has the potential to address local and global issues that women face in and outside of the hospital.[113] Faith-based institutions might utilize the findings in this report to focus on the significance of identifying spiritual distress in antepartum women. A need exists for additional theological and biblical study about spiritual distress among antepartum patients. Offering renewed hope in the midst of their despair can enhance a Christian leader's relationship with these women.

This research might serve as an evangelistic outreach tool for mothers seeking answers to the problematic questions prevalent to the needs of antepartum women. Heightened spiritual support in the antepartum world may reveal the need to pay closer attention to these "ladies-in-waiting." Brochures, pamphlets, or fliers with research results reported in this paper might be helpful information for doctor's offices, clinics, and women's conferences. These implications would support the need for an ongoing conversation about a population of women who need a particular nine-months-or-less level of spiritual support. Harold Koenig addresses the need to, "examine humans improved changes in the physical body... during religious services (public or private), which include prayer, singing of religious hymns, and other rituals."[114]

113 References to my personal history are found in *Implications for Contemporary Ministry*, Chapter 5.
114 Koenig, Spirituality and Health Research, 56.

Koenig concludes that, in the United States, over 40 percent of faith-based believers involve themselves in these activities once a week. Religion and spiritual health or spirituality (R/S) reveals fewer common health problems among those who are more inclined to religion and spirituality.[115] This chaplain's hope is that the findings of this study will be supported to hospital chaplains as they help antepartum patients find hope during their periods of spiritual distress. The difficulty in determining a "one size fits all" spiritual distress measurement tool for antepartum patient care rests in the multiplicity of prenatal patients' diverse needs. The scope can be broader than the single challenge of the need for mandatory bed rest. A multitude of factors also exist. Consider additional considerations to support antepartum women that the chaplain has observed over the years.[116]

BIOGRAPHICAL, CHURCH, AND VOCATIONAL HISTORY FOR FUTURE MINISTRY APPLICATIONS

An unexpected result of this research project has prompted a reflection on the early years of my private, professional experiences and service regarding young expectant mothers and their families. The discovery was prompted by the thought that additional and contributing attributes may provide some additional information that will contribute to a more comprehensive publication. The new information might assist others in understanding the breadth and depth of my interest in providing support to antepartum women.

FAMILY HISTORY: INTRODUCTION INTO THE ANTEPARTUM WORLD

My family history, upon reflection, has a strong spiritual connection to the beginnings of my enlightenment about the needs of antepartum women. Maternal relationships are essential in the lives

---

115 Ibid.
116 This entire section details past experiences with antepartum women.

of prenatal patients in the hospital. The following event supports the warm connection mothers have with their unborn babies. The experience would evolve into a spiritual connection to this project for me. My mother lived in the family homestead with her mother (my grandmother), the rest of the family, including my father, three older children, and other family members.

Spousal support was also unique when my mother was in an antenatal state. She carried a baby who weighed in at birth at 14 pounds and 10 ounces. She needed help from her support system; her husband (my father), remained a pillar of strength throughout the pregnancy. One sister's account was that Mom was in labor for five days. My older sister recalls our father preparing coffee and sweetbreads for the many doctors who decided to come to care for the patient in her home, prior to the birth of the baby. It was reported that the doctors provided ongoing care to the patient for four days. The baby was at last delivered in an area hospital. My mother's faith and tenacity also contributed to the health and wellness of both mother and baby. She would also detail her feelings about a nearby clergy neighbor and friend who encouraged her in her "walk of faith." The significance for contemporary ministry, in this way, reflects the essentials for maintaining a strong, church, community, and family ties during emergent situations in pregnancy. A chaplain can be made aware that there are other reliable avenues of spiritual support surrounding the patient. Pastoral Care can be on-going in the life of the patient. Hospital chaplaincy is unique in that it may serve as an extension to many facets of their faith-based support in the community.

Vocational History/The Value of School and Community Support for Unwed and Married Teens

The early teaching years, immediately following university education, sets the stage for my initial journey with antepartum patients.

In addition to my school vocational history, I also served as a church youth leader. An additional contemporary component to this paper may broaden the scope of this project. The present study focuses on Baylor Hospital's pre-term mothers in hospital ministry. A further consideration, however, for the health of antepartum patients begins with excellent home support and consistent prenatal care.

I had the opportunity during my early teaching years to support the work of the school Guidance Department with teacher team support groups for teens expecting babies. The stories of these young mothers revealed a long list of considerations not covered in the body of this paper.[117] In those days, some students were active church members who expressed reservations about attending church during their pregnancies. The school, in this same venue, provided excellent support for many young expectant women. The school provided, in-school daycare centers, financed night school (GED classes for those nearing graduation), and helped with transportation to clinical appointments. After teacher counseling sessions, many young mothers sought additional counseling from their home churches and their pastors. The school program was funded by a government agency; an advantage that sometimes exists with the present twenty-first-century economy.[118]

I envision enlightening churches, pastors, laypersons, family members, community organizations, and other support groups about some of the basic needs of prenatal women. My early vocational history connects to this project in many ways. Having taught

---

117 The study of more themes might broaden the insights of a variety of healthcare institutions. Community health-fares, community clinics, mid-wife practitioners, and other institutions might benefit from the scope of this research.
118 BUMC supports the Life Design Program for young teen expectant, mothers in collaboration with Buckner International. The Transition School in my past also provided off campus curriculum classes that ensured subsequent graduations in individual teens' area high schools (the home schools they were to which they were formally enrolled.

school for eight years in Virginia, at the alternative school and two elementary schools, I became interested in, and was exposed to the essentials of family and community support systems in the lives of antepartum mothers. Community Centers, Churches, Schools, Area Healthcare facilities, and other institutions, could partner together to develop like models of support.

More Support Ministry/Vocational History that Influences a Contemporary Model of Care for Antepartum Patients

The following details might shed more light on a renewed direction of spiritual support to antepartum women. My early experiences took place in the late 1970s and the early 1980s.[119] My early experiences as a teacher at the Transition School (an alternative high school located in Norfolk, Virginia) introduced me to a world of young women with a broad list of spiritual needs.[120] While the needs of young male students were also addressed at this high school institution, many students were unwed mothers with children, while others were married with children. One might think that the differences in the needs of these students might be insufficient to support the claims of this project. The extreme significance of the

---

119 The Transition School formed just after the Brown vs. Brown Board of Education case ensued, when changes took place in Virginia's de-segregation legislation laws. Many high schools experienced racial tensions that affected high school student life from a variety of ethnicities and income levels. Sponsored by Title I, the educational goals of the school were positioned to provide an alternative school that would address the socio-economic needs of the students who were not prepared for the transition. Many others considered the school to be a "last chance" school. Thomas Newby, the first principal at the school, completed a Ph.D. about his work with a program that addressed the needs of students at a strategic time when the integration of schools began. The connection for this project lies in the many opportunities team teachers provided in educational counseling sessions to listen to the concerns of unwed mothers, whose children received in-school child-care and worked with counselors to help support student's job searches through the school guidance department.
120 The alternative school supported students for a decade; the graduates completed their high school diplomas at their respective schools, obtained GED's or transitioned to gainful employment during and after completing high school.

two vocational and ministerial experiences, among others, form a complete picture.

I took notice about how the young women demonstrated a child-like faith during the life experiences and challenging odds against them. The school was designed to ensure that students would complete their high school training with renewed life and job skills. Employees in the town partnered with the school system and provided part-time and full-time employment for these students. Since a few of the mothers were expecting babies, the school program made it possible for them to continue their education on a contractual basis that allowed maternity leave, completing assignments at home, and half workdays. I observed the steady faith and support of these students' parents and grandparents. The Norfolk Public School System must also be commended for their support of these "last chance" students. These students would be able to graduate later from their respective high schools with dignity. Mothers who delivered babies before graduation were given the opportunity to walk down the aisles at graduation in their respective public high schools, while few of their fellow students were aware of their struggles.

The Norfolk school board selected the teachers at the Transition School from area high schools, specifically choosing those who were certified teachers from the military, trained high school counselors, and other professionals.[121] In reflection, the essentials of teamwork in that educational setting would transform into the viable multi-disciplinary teamwork needed to support antepartum mothers at BUMC. Just as the needs of unwed mothers and families in my past were supported by their faith communities, counselors,

---

121 The Transition School was also supported by the Norfolk Public School System; a government, Magnet, program established in 1972. High School Principals; Thomas Newby, Theodore Little, and John Osteen maintained an exceptional and alternative academic program for alternative students; promoting academic excellence. Their collective visions of support for students were noteworthy.

teachers, and families, so the team huddles demonstrated a solid multi-disciplinary and multi-faceted voice of support for antepartum mothers. The four major high schools were extremely involved in supporting these transitional students, as the temporary transfer of students needed supportive networks.

The Transition School was where I experienced the need for family and church support with the teens under my tutelage. During parent and teacher conferences, I saw first-hand how much family and faith-based institutions provided the support needed during family crises. Support groups through community health initiatives, area churches, and the School Guidance Department enlisted these institutions' help to assist unwed mothers throughout their difficult journeys. Students from all ethnicities and economic backgrounds experienced the same unfortunate situations that surrounded the new beginnings of young families. Many students who graduated high school from their home high schools often matriculated onto college, obviously benefitting from the support they received from the Transition School.

The experiences with these young women prepared me for work within the hospital culture. While the populations in schools and hospitals are different, the exposure and spiritual needs for both seemed to address the plight of pre-term women. One common denominator for this chaplain was the faith-based references that were consistently uttered by both the teens and those resting in the hospital.[122] In considering implications for furthering the aspects of this project, many community institutions and enterprises might find this study useful for supporting women and others with those

---

122 A few teens, both in the early vocational history at the Transition School and the current hospital culture at Baylor, reflect the teen's practice of reading the Bible. Many were raised by Christian mothers and grandmothers who maintain their love for the church, current church hymns, and a deep and abiding faith in Christ.

perplexing hard cases that are present in our churches, communities, and in other programs in the healthcare profession.

My early vocation had been that of an Art Educator at the Transition School. The school curriculum granted me the opportunity to teach faith-based art history on the high school level among other curriculum-oriented art classes.[123] In reflection, the art education background was useful in the chaplain residents' expressions of the theological themes mentioned in chapter 3. The art framework would also come into play in my Master's Level Thesis that included a theological, church, and faith-based Cartoon Companion.[124]

Also helpful was my church training as a young adult youth minister, Sunday school teacher, and Vacation Bible School teacher after graduating college at Bank Street Baptist Church in Norfolk, Virginia. The joy experienced in the church youth ministry was exceptional, yet I also recall feelings of inadequacy in relating to the young adults who seemed to drift away from church attendance. The balance came when opportunities for service came with youth speaking engagements, speaking for college Bible study groups, and Baptist denominational Vacation Bible School Training sessions.[125]

The scope of this project may have some connection to how I learned successful and helpful ways to connect with young women who craved improved spiritual direction. Many students faced

---

123 The role of art educator at the Transition School, afforded the opportunity to teach faith-based art history, among other high school curriculum-oriented art classes. Art projects often emulated periods in history that reflected depictions of biblical characters, and biblical subjects ranging from the fourteenth century to the present. Field trips to area and tri-city museums provided opportunities to present faith-based visuals and stories to students.

124 Master of Arts in Communication in the School of Educational Ministries; Southwestern Baptist Theological Seminary in Fort Worth, Texas, 2004.

125 Youth Ministry Leadership Opportunities at Eagle Eyrie Baptist Conference Center in Lynchburg, VA, Ridgecrest Baptist Conference Center in Ashville, North, Carolina, Baptist Student Ministry (BSM) One Night Fellowship Opportunities at The University of Richmond, and Virginia Commonwealth University, both in Richmond VA. Also served in the Evening Fellowship Opportunities in BSM at Old Dominion University in Norfolk, VA, and Hampton University in Hampton, VA.

spiritual trials and sought ways to cope with relational difficulties. I was single during those formative years. Many other youth ministries across the states of Texas and Virginia produced great similarities between the cities and rural communities. Youth ministries continued to flourish in those days.

Later, in 1981, I married and continued to discover yet another profound direction in my vocation in Virginia. I taught in a one-class-per-grade-level, red-brick elementary schoolhouse in Doswell, Virginia, as well as teaching at a regular elementary school with two or three classes per grade level in another city. It was at these elementary schools that I witnessed other family systems.

Throughout that year, I discovered first-hand the importance of shaping the lives of elementary-age children who would assist me in learning the value of steady faith-based family living. Observing quality, rural education at the two elementary schools provided strong models for Christian family life. The principals, teachers, and parents of children were an amazing group of people, modeling the value of teamwork and ethical, Christian leadership. This was the beginning of growth for me as it relates to this project because, by the end of the school year, I was expecting our first child. The transition from being a working woman to a stay-at-home mother would be an identifiable experience that is familiar to the new antepartum mothers in the hospital. While I was not in a state of distress, or on mandatory bed rest, carrying a child was and is helpful to an understanding of the nature of antepartum mothers.

The connection for me was the reality that my family was one-hundred miles away, while I was coping with my husband's job schedule, which required a lot of travel. At intervals, both of our mothers and siblings visited to provide support. Additionally, the church community and friends provided the necessary support system that was needed. The blessings came when I began to travel with my husband extensively during those safe months. Now, when I observe antepartum mothers with little-to-no support, I clearly recall the gratitude I felt for my surrounding family and church support system. For this reason, I believe my past experiences have assisted in moving forward with this project.

The chance to serve at Baylor again in 2013 was an opportunity of a lifetime. While I may forget the names and faces of many of these mothers over the years, I have great comfort in knowing that MCH chaplains will continue to provide quality health care to these women.

Increasing teen pregnancies and prenatal care issues are important. All pastoral care healthcare providers must continue to upgrade the discovery of the diverse needs of antepartum women. Chaplains might consider addressing the supportive roles of family members, detailing the significance of addressing "family first," in a future publication. Pre-term mothers and their families may benefit from some form of ethical dialogue about fidelity in marriage. Others may be informed with Christian based reading about the ethics in the institution of marriage and related family relationships, as it relates to the health and wellbeing of antepartum mothers.

The hospital portion of the literature might delve into a woman's spiritual and prenatal needs that focus on monitoring visitations by family, church members, friends, spouses, and small children. Chaplains might offer suggestions for family and guests to consider during visitation. Guests might also consider food restrictions, quieter verbal communications, or consider stepping out in the hall when the baby's heart is being monitored. A pamphlet of this nature will suggest ways to provide compassionate care to mothers-to-be. Some intentionality can also be exercised in other aspects of patient visitation. There might be a concerted effort on the part of family, friends, and other visitors, to keep conversations low-key, away from difficult subjects, and to time shorter visits during scheduled nap times.

Concluding Thoughts Concerning Contemporary Ministry

In conclusion, after the results of the on-line surveys were completed for this project, one may approach the topic of ministry to antepartum women in a renewed light. The results of the surveys may also prompt the writing of a book or pamphlet that would serve patients well. Informative and inspirational language could be presented in a series of pamphlets that address current topics in the field of spiritually distressed prenatal mothers. The theological themes could be expanded to begin a new work; establishing spiritual distress with additional theological themes. A book or pamphlet sequel to this project also might serve patients better who do not want to be labeled as spiritually distressed patients. Chaplains might better address antepartum mothers' medical states by demonstrating skill in listening to the needs of patients with a non-anxious presence. The goal for chaplains will be upgraded to provide helpful and significant support from chaplains whose patients show no evidence of spiritual distress.

The hospital chaplain might also consider providing a more generic book or flyer for a vast arena of other institutions and community facilities. Readers would be introduced and directed to the impact of the image of God, faith, hope, and suffering to patients and their healthcare providers. A published journal article or book may usher in a definitive and positive impact on existing community efforts for antepartum patients. The generic title of a possible book or pamphlet of this nature might also attract the interests of antepartum patients. Healthcare providers might also be prompted to read and consider unique ways to address the basic needs of antepartum patients from a different perspective. Many providers

and institutions might learn or glean from helpful perspectives presented in such a publication. A broad and general "good read" might
generate interest from couples who have decided to choose mid-
wives to deliver their babies. Again, caution would be used in clari-
fying the point that such a publication would not emphasize medical
terminology but would lean more toward spiritual support to antepartum patients. Supportive and professional support will, however,
be solicited by the chaplain from faith-based healthcare providers.

The antepartum mother, in general, may also benefit from a
pamphlet, distinctive to the unique and spiritual needs of the mother-to-be and her growing infant. I, therefore, propose the development of a manual that would detail the roles of those providing care
to antepartum women. Such a manual would be a resource for pastors, church staff, laypersons, and family members, (such as spouses, parents, siblings, and children), as they support antepartum
women. Through the information provided in the manual, professionals and family members might explore the need for intentional,
compassionate language needed on patient visitations. Patient supporters might consider the model Jesus demonstrated in the Bible
attributed to Christ's love, compassion, and humility.

Patients need spiritual support that reflects the humanity Christ
showed to those in need. In this way, pastors and laypersons will
better assess the needs of patients. The benefits for providers will
move them toward improved listening and attending skills. Brief "to
do" lists will provide suggestions for better engagement by close
friends and family members of patients, during those moments of
medical challenge. Leaving toddler children with mothers on bedrest over long periods, for example, might cause medical complications. Curtailing stressful conversations would be another example
of visitations that reflect intentional care for the whole person of
the antenatal mother. The possibility of presenting a secular and a

Christian publication might assist the healthcare industry and the masses about the needs of antepartum patients as well as other patients who might benefit from the inferences and the actual research expressed in the "hidden" five theological themes. An additional consideration might include several different theological themes that were not researched in this project.

A faith-based Christian book or pamphlet might also serve Christians and those who would believe in the Gospel message. Individuals and institutions might be prompted to utilize the five themes described in this paper, inpatient visitations. The research might inform the masses about the unique experiences of an antepartum mother. The project itself could be published as a theological and biblical presentation. The general essence of such a book would address the spiritual needs of patients from a Christian perspective. As explained earlier, many other theological themes could be introduced. A theology of "family first," might serve the likes of all family members in the life of patients, including in-laws and grandparents. Chaplains, pastors, and church laypersons might learn to merge their goals to the betterment of patients.

Future publications might include more subjects that relate to marriage, family, and informative presentations about child-care and other family-specific medical interests. Within a Christian context, the additional food for thought would provide biblical aspects for consideration. Addressing general prognoses about pre-term medical conditions could be presented in a Christian context. The broader subjects might relate to antepartum mothers including detailed topics about what to expect with the birth of pre-term babies. Examples might include healing words of spiritual support to mothers who volunteer information about a possible anomaly or problem the baby is expected to have.

Other significant theological themes were not researched or addressed in this paper. Additional themes might enhance the way chaplains provide care to antepartum women. An extended presentation would lean heavily on a publication that would affirm and educate the masses about antepartum women. A revised presentation would add excerpts from peer-reviewed articles that address spiritual distress in antepartum patients.

Since there has been no singular and established definition of spiritual distress across hospital disciplines, the scope of the project may need adjustment. Perhaps we might render more thought on how to determine spiritual distress in antepartum patients. An additional perspective might suggest individual theological terms and pre-suppositions develop a more comprehensive approach to the difficult subject of spiritual distress. In other words, the individual theological themes would stand alone. In this way the themes could address independent research on each topic rather than clumping themes together to reflect a general definition of spiritual distress.

At Baylor Hospital, the chaplain might make available to patients, individual flyers, and pamphlets at the disposal of patients in the Antepartum Family Room. Current subject headings might attract mothers-to-be to read insightful Bible-based information. The reading material would directly apply to marriage and family issues. These brochures will be informational and presented from a Christian perspective. Patients might be informed about such things as the sacred commitment in institution of marriage, the theology of, "family first," fidelity in marriage, best spiritual support practices for teen mothers, and other current topics.

I recall attending a wedding by a French African couple who were expecting to have their NICU baby in a couple of months. The wedding took place in the foyer on one of the top, non-patient room floors at Baylor. The bride was beautiful as family members and friends gathered from near and far to attend the wedding. A Dallas Justice-of-the-Peace performed the ceremony. The groom was adorned with a nice tuxedo. No food was served, and only two witnesses stood with the couple, but the event demonstrated hope. Most of the guests spoke in French and seemed pleased by the chaplain's presence. Artificial floral arrangements were already in the room, and the couple took full advantage of the scenery. It dawned on me that the pre-term mothers who hold on to hope have opportunities despite the odds. The beauty of the wedding sums up the themes in this project. Following one's dreams and making perfect choices may result in significant dialogue between patients and chaplains.

The five theological themes, among others, present many opportunities for growth in patients, and chaplain residents.[126] I hope each participant had the opportunity to internalize their personal theological perspectives in this study. My prayer is that antepartum patients seek to discover more elements of hope amid suffering. There is divine hope in God in the salvation work of *Jesus, The Suffering Servant*. God suffers with believers. Christ walks with and listens to believers who are genuinely formed in his image. Past, present, and future respect for the church sustains and encourages believers in the midst of their separation from weekly church attendance. The eschatological hope that ushers in Christ's appearing comforts and inspires believers to trust in God in spite of spiritual and physical hindrances.[127]

Again, it is my prayer that each theological theme flyer positively inspired others. Christ continuously walks into antepartum

126 The themes are detailed in Chapter 3, "Theological Reflection." The themes were selected out of a list of theological themes based on a compilation of definitions on spiritual distress. See footnote number 24.
127 My husband and I hold membership at "The Exciting Singing Hills Baptist Church" in Dallas, TX. Dr. Howard E. Anderson, Sr., pastor. I have served as a coach in Children's Church, served in the Grief Ministry and enjoy Sunday School.

patient rooms. The Holy Spirit continues to guide inspired chaplain residents. God will resonate within my heart continued concern for the spiritual plight of antepartum patients. The literature that is bound to grow from this project would be approved by Baylor's upper management to ensure that the language and presentation would support the hospital's mission and message. The possibilities and resources for such a work are endless. Just as no biblical record exists of an Acts 29, this writer anticipates that other believers might find valuable treasures in the hearts and minds of pastoral care providers (themselves) to fine-tune their call with the people of God whom they have been assigned to spiritually support.

The love of God, in the name of Christ, in the power of the Holy Spirit, gives antepartum mothers a hope that is the already-and-the-not-yet. Experiencing the unknown is tempered well when patients feel spiritually supported by chaplains who sense that patients seek a deeper dialogue in Christ. With the support of spiritually prepared chaplains, patients consider the significance of the Gospel message. Compassionate pastoral care providers can move from a place of spiritual uneasiness to a place of respite peace.

To summarize the claim in this project, looking at "the significance of pastoral support in addressing spiritual distress in antepartum patients,"[128] the results are astounding. The surprise element came when the results of the on-line survey produced no significant changes from the "two-tailed t-test measuring tool," that calibrated the results of the on-line surveys. The controlled visitations were intended to support the new chaplain residents with antepartum patients, patients to whom they were not accustomed to visiting. Future projects may serve patients better when controlled visits are not a part of the plan.[129]

128 The title of this project.
129 In the earlier class sessions, the project director selected patient and chaplain resident visitation appointments. Unplanned visitations on the floors may have produced more authentic dialogues through prayer and

The project accomplished many things as antepartum patients might now be better understood. Significant theological themes were addressed in the life of antepartum patients. The spiritual connections and dialogues by chaplains with antepartum patients were informative. A presentation of additional themes might produce a better spiritual distress definition.[130] There were no significant changes in the scoring of pre and post on-line surveys by chaplains in this project, and I was grateful that the goals were accomplished. More work is needed to support the antepartum "ladies in waiting." Prenatal women deserve the utmost pastoral care from a God-breathed mode of spiritual support.

There is a theology of a strong ministry of presence, for lonely, sad, confused, sick, desperate for comfort in thinking about their babies' conditions, and lack of walking freedom for various antepartum patients. The significance of pastoral support lies in the forward movement of pastoral care providers. Chaplains comfort others with caring dialogue and compassionate listening skills to the needs of patients. Patients need all the spiritual support that they are capable of receiving on a pastoral visit. Though difficult to master, the significance lies in a forward Christ-like movement that seeks to imitate Christ's perfect love. With pastoral skill, sincerity, and spiritual gentility, a chaplain's single desire is to provide an ideal mode of spiritual support to distressed patients. Patients need direction and help in figuring the tough situations they find themselves. Family members, friends, healthcare providers, and even chaplains must store more room for spiritual growth within themselves. Antepartum patients might need a multiplicity of theological themes to consider. The

in-the-moment and spirit led pastoral support. See Chapter 2, "General Project Summary, Meeting Six."

130 As detailed in the introduction; The definition of spiritual distress in this paper is a disruption in the life principle that pervades a person's entire being that integrates and transcends one's biological . . . nature; a form of suffering related to the impaired ability to experience meaning in life through connections with self, others, the world, or a superior being.

themes may be different from the way the mother is approaching her illness in comparison to the medical condition of her forming baby. In conclusion, the conversation I embraced was a collective read from theologians and Bible scholars who pointed this project in a God-ward direction.

An exhaustive list of related antepartum subjects and situations might merge with the goals of this project. The educational program experienced might produce a significant record in addition to that of the hospital culture: Subjects unexplored topics such as family and peer shame, personal guilt, incest, rape reasons for Child Protective Service investigations, court-related issues, adoption, feelings of spiritual alienation, separation from support systems, significant family or friend loss of life, other family illnesses, unable to maintain a comfortable family life, loss of friends, unable to participate in favorite sports or other hobbies and extra, curricular activities, disconnected from school environment or special interest groups or clubs, and ridicule from church members and church friends. I close with a simple message to antepartum mothers

Ode to an Antenatal Mother

Please let us know when you want to rest,
For you and your baby deserve less stress.
You are already standing the test;
As you do your best.
To see God in it
Where you fit
Into his plan
Amen?
Don't elope
Hope
Let us in
No ostrich sand
Or in just a little while;
We'll see your engaging smile.
One day you may just shed a tear,
Or try telling us your doubts or fears.
You just hold on, with a glorious view of the eschaton.
And thank Jesus, the true champion of love as your perfect race is run
In Christ's Image, your formation and spirituality improves
As you relish memories of the Church, the Good News!
Continue your walk of faith, soon theologies to embrace.
With you, hope in God, Creation, the Fall and the tree
Know that you and your baby are sincerely loved
From the Master above
So don't go away
No AMA today
Stay.
Pray.

The Author's Personal Note: A Hope for the Generations

The broader significance of this book reflects the support systems needed for antepartum mothers. Prenatal care, church and community involvement, the family, healthcare facilities, and support organizations that begin a need-based roll call. The antepartum mother literally blesses her coming generation.

Families are strengthened as optimal care of a growing baby is prioritized. If we could envision the life span of a prenatal baby until her adulthood, many amazing stories would have taken place. I call your attention to the last photograph in this book. I am flinging my hands up in a joyous celebration. I am grateful that you have read this book. My heartfelt sentiment is to relay a message of hope for the plight of the antepartum journey. The bigger picture points to a big world out there that pays attention to their needs. Or it could just be you, an antepartum mother who becomes an agent and a blessing for the generations to come.

There is victorious hope, despite the obstacles. With ongoing support systems during pregnancy, one's life story has a chance to blossom. All of the personal photographs in this book are but a model that pale to the rainbow blueprints other pre-term mothers will show others. They can opt to fill in the blanks of their own spiritual journeys with eschatological hope!

Perhaps you, the church triumphant, community services, family, or friends, will continue to embrace this wonderful population of women world-wide and pay attention to their antepartum needs. If you are an antepartum woman, I say pass it on, embrace your beauty in Christ Jesus! Whatever the outcomes, rallying we can help others find "triumphant hope in the midst of despair."

APPENDIX A

Online Surveys[131]

Chaplains' Responses on Antepartum Unit

Ten Question On-Line Survey Questions given to the chaplain residents:

Q1 I want a visit to go as quickly as possible.

Q2 I am intentional about heightened listening with the patient.

Q3 I am fully aware when the patient wants me to help her in her distress.

---

131 For clarification, the numeric figures for the on-line surveys included the results of the combined scores of the project director as well as those of the chaplain residents, totaling seven responses. The initial composite number should have been eight, including the project director's scores. However, the report is authentic, as some students—for whatever reason—missed one weekly completion of the on-line survey. An even scoring based on the figures balanced the results of the on-line surveys. Thus, the margin of error in the scores is minimal, as it was difficult to ascertain the persons who did not complete the surveys.

Q4 I am fully aware when the patient posits that this is not a good time for a visit.

Q5 I am not personally offended if the patient does not want to see a chaplain.

Q6 I respect a healthcare provider's assessment that the patient is not up for a visit.

Q7 I recognize the significance of my visit and the patient's spirituality.

Q8 I am comfortable listening to the spiritual distress of the patient.

Q9 I admit my own discomfort in listening to the spiritual distress of this patient.

APPENDIX B

The Survey Results

PAIRED TWO-TAILED T-TEST [132]

The numbers in the t-test suggest the standard by which a scale is measured. The scores in this test align with a consistency that measured the Pre-and Post-Surveys that were presented to chaplain residents in this study. The surveys were presented to the seven Clinical Pastoral Education chaplain resident participants at the beginning, throughout, and at the end of the training classes to arrive at some form of measurement that would reflect patient visitations before, during, and after receiving the training. The results indicate the level of care and pastoral support provided to a variety of patients after receiving the training. The results of the surveys reflect

---

132 Gratitude to Clay Price, who is retired from the Baptist General Convention of Texas, and whose review and insights were appreciated in the resulting calibrations over the pre- and post-surveys used in this project. The results are posted at the end of this description. The suggested theological, educational, and ministerial insights are entered based on Clay Prices' overall conclusion that the results may be better explained by an alternative use of logic.

an outcrop of certain factors. The studies addressed the stress (spiritual distress) or comfort levels in their role as chaplains in their care of antepartum patients. The results provided a consistency that was tallied before and after a group of chaplains received training from the project director. The goal of the t-test was to determine whether the attitudes or feelings changed significantly after the training. This type of study is called a paired sample, and the t-statistic was used to determine whether the before and after values were significantly different.

The t-test was begun with a null hypothesis: The final meaning and conclusion posit that there was no significant difference between the before and after scores. The average difference of pre- and post-scores for all the participants in the survey, therefore resulted in a "0" range. Each of the ten survey items was independent of one another, so the overall score presents the overall data with ten items separately scored, each with their own t-stats. In most studies the t-stat is typically used for measuring continuous values like weight or height, but it can be used for discrete values from Likert scales (that approximate continuous values). The latter was used in this project. The t-test is a statistic that can be used to determine if there is a statistical difference between two values in a setting where the values are measured before and after some treatment or training or intervention. The formula by which the test was measured, in this case reflect the many tools that calculated each value. The t-test was used as a function for paired two-tailed samples that can be found in the Excel Data Analysis tools.

A separate worksheet was provided for each of the ten survey items. Looking at the tab for Q1, the left side of the worksheet shows the scores for the seven participants from their pre- and post-test surveys. The mean (average) score is at the bottom of the table. In the pre-test the seven participants averaged 2.429 as their response to the item *I want a visit to go as quickly as possible*. The mean score is close to 2 which means they tended to agree with the statement. In the post-test their mean score was 5.429 which is close to 5, meaning they now tended to disagree with the statement. Logically, there was a significant change in this item. Something happened that made them no longer feel that visits should go quickly. We would expect the difference in scores to be significant, and the t-stat confirms it.

The t-stat value was -9.72111 (cell H12). It has a negative value because the pre-score was subtracted from the post-score. If the post-score had been deducted from the pre-score, the t-stat would have been a positive 9.72111. This process is therefore referred to as a two-tailed test because the statistic can be determined either way.

In creating the statistic .05 (5%) was used as the cutoff value for the probability that there was no statistical difference in the pre and post scores. Two values that tell us what we want to know. The first (cell H15) is the probability from the equation for the scores related to Q1. P is .00006804 which is much, much lower than .05. There was less than a 5% chance that the null hypothesis was true. Put another way, we say we are 95% sure that the difference was not due to chance or random variation.

The second value that also confirms statistical difference is the "t Critical two-tail" value in cell H16. That value is 2.4469 which tells us our t-stat must be higher than this to indicate a statistical difference in scores. The results in running this two-tailed test reveal that t Critical and can also be -2.4469 (so if our t-stat is negative, it has to be lower than -2.4469 to be significant). Observed is (above) that our t-stat is -9.72111 and is clearly lower than -2.4469.

The manual measurement on the bar graph shows that the Excel formula generated the exact same t-stat. Below the manual calculation posits a normal distribution graph of t-stats. The shaded "tails" on the left and right side of the graph show a t-stat that is either higher than the 2.4469 on the right or lower than the -2.4469 on the left in order to reject the null hypothesis that the difference in scores are caused by chance or random variation.

The other tabs, Q2 to Q10, show the results of the equations, observing the values in cells H12 and H15 and H16 to determine whether there is statistical difference between the pre and post scores on each item. The two items which calibrated no statistical differences are as follows: The first is Q4 that resulted in a rare situation where the t-stat cannot be calculated because the formula ends up with a 0 for the divisor, as shown in the manual calculation at the bottom of the table. In this case one may turn to logic. The seven participants agreed (mean score was 2.285) they "were fully aware when the patient posits it is not a good time to visit" before they took the training. After the training, their agreement with the statement was closer to strongly agree (mean score 1.286). Their awareness improved a little, but it was pretty strong at the start. A statistical difference may or may not exist.

The t-stat for Q6 was 2.1213, and the P-value was .078. This indicates there was not a statistical difference in the pre and post scores. A look at the mean scores becomes logical. Before the training, the participants slightly agreed they "respected the healthcare provider's assessment that a patient was not up for a visit" (mean score 3.428). After the training they tended to feel slightly better about the healthcare provider's assessment (mean score 3.000). Now that it has been ascertained whether or not each item yielded a significant change from the pre to post-test surveys, the question is asked, "Did the training make a difference, or could there have been some other variables that contributed to the difference?" There is an added bar chart on worksheet "Sheet1" starting in cell B34. It shows the mean scores for the pre and post-test surveys for each of the 10 survey items. The differences in the scores are observed here. There is very little difference for Q6 and with limited statistical difference for pre and post scores on this item. Q7 is something of a surprise because the difference was significant, and the scores are very similar to Q4 (where the formula could not be computed). Even though the Q7 pre and post were statistically different, there was really only a minimal change among the participants in their feeling that they "recognize the significance of their visits and the patient's spirituality" (mean score from 2.143 to 1.286). One explanation might be the other side of the statistical data. The results reflect a statistical difference between the actual question or the measurement; and the change remains relatively small. Logic may serve this study well.[133] It is impossible to account for all variables but perhaps there might be something that occurred that could have affected all of the participants. In this research the question is asked, "What else could have contributed to these results? The following may apply:

THEOLOGICAL, SPIRITUAL AND EDUCATIONAL DIMENSIONS RELATED TO THIS STUDY

1. The Pre and Post-Surveys in this study were not adequate in determining levels of spiritual distress patients in antepartum patients for chaplain residents. An alternative measurement tool may therefore better serve antepartum patients who are experiencing spiritual distress.

2. The theological themes in this paper were not exhaustive enough to address the theological implications in this paper.

3. The theological aptitudes of patients were not adequately assessed by chaplains.

---

133 A position quoted by Clay Price.

4. Improved theological and biblical study on the existing themes addressed in this paper.

5. Another testing instrument calibrating the results of ante-partum patients who have admitted elements of spiritual distress; may produce a truer picture of spiritually distressed pre-term mothers.

6. This study took place seven months of a twelve-month pro-gram of competency training. Multiple training didactics in Clinical Pastoral Education (CPE) may have demonstrated learned pastoral skill, in patient visitations by chaplain res-idents five months prior to the closing of their training at Level I CPE.

7. The study may have been a controlled a study that may have limited the selection of patients based on the project direc-tor's hand-picked selection of patients for chaplain residents.

8. Chaplains might discover that many antepartum patients do not determine that their own hospital stays in the hospital are spiritually distressful.

9. Antepartum patients may not feel comfortable discussing spiritual distress with chaplain residents and may have pre-ferred to remain positive in their conversations about them-selves or their coming babies.

10. Chaplain residents' provision of care to faith-based pa-tients might reflect the patients' minimal biblical interest in

discussing spiritual distress in comparison to their medical conditions in the moment.

11. Chaplain residents may normalize an antepartum patient's spirituality based on the biblical text: "Verily, I say unto you, that you shall weep and lament, but the world will rejoice and you will be sorrowful, but your sorrow will be turned into joy. A woman when she is in travail has sorrow, because her hour is come: but as soon as she is delivered of the child, she remembers no more the anguish, for joy that a man is born into the world. And you now therefore have sorrow: but I will see you again, and your heart will rejoice, and your joy no man takes from you" (John 16:20-22).

12. Chaplain residents successfully inspired patients with the Theological Themes in the Encouragement Flyers during this study. The flyers might have resonated with the imbedded theologies of faith based chaplains as well as the patients. The medical conditions surrounding their hospital stays might have had more weight in the moment than patient's spiritual dialogues about their feelings of spiritual distress.

13. Testimonials from chaplain residents revealed their personal spiritual healing after the five theological themes were presented by the project director.

14. The project director noticed improved pastoral support by the chaplain residents throughout the duration of the projects.

15. The pre and post surveys in this project might serve as an unrealistic approach toward addressing spiritual distress.

16. There may exist a far-reaching, and general assumption that all antepartum patients from the chaplain's perspective, are experiencing similar levels of spiritual distress; that needs adjustment.

17. In reflection, this paper focused on the techniques needed in pastoral support to antepartum patients. The perspective might be amply adjusted to less generalizations. Spiritual distress can be determined at best with individual cases. This paper might have made the premature assumption that all antepartum patients are spiritually distressed.

18. An alternative measuring tool might apply after patients, staff and other healthcare providers have determined that spiritual distress is a indeed a factor with select patients.

19. Consider utilizing more support from the healthcare team who support faith-based initiatives.

20. One might consider the needs of patients in stressful situations to focus more on the urgency of spiritual needs, while not downplaying the theological maturity some of patients.

21. The chaplain could develop a more efficient way to meet with patients in less than ten minutes of their requests.

22. The chaplain might upgrade their evangelistic efforts for un-churched patients.

APPENDIX E

Creative Literature from a Resident

"CHILDREN'S CHAPLAIN"
BY TOWNLEY BARNES MCGIFFERT

running on empty,
pushing prayers;
soft pedaling God,
the overwhelming infinite —
intimate trauma of belief.

Jesus, save this child—
don't let me give false hope—
you who were once a homeless babe,
a donkey for a midwife,
give birth to faith again
for this holy family.

they don't want me near,
they think my presence means death is here;

it stings to be misunderstood.
"what are your alternatives?"
I want to ask
"stainless nihilism or nowness-with-spirit?"

often the forced options of life sting.
choose love if you can.
doors slam and bang in the halls
of the holy hurried clinic
I bed down annoyed,
alone with the echoes of hope.[134]

The chaplain residents were asked to name three feelings with which they might identify as they read this writer's poem. The residents were asked to detail examples they observed in prior visits with any patient. The residents were instructed to do the following: On the paper provided, compose a short poem about an experience you have had with an antepartum patient, while paying close attention to observing notable spiritual distress indicators with antepartum patients or families. They are also asked to detail how they have experienced any of the theological themes from the five theological themes they have experienced in their personal journeys:

ACTIVITY

Identify with one or more of the words presented in the encouragement flyers with a brief description about how one can connect with the word, _____:

---

134 Townley Barnes McGiffert, Children's Chaplain. Journal of Pastoral Care and Counseling (Summer 2002), 196. McGiffert wrote this poem during his chaplain residency at Emory Healthcare in Atlanta, GA.

APPENDIX F

A Spiritual Distress Instrument[135]

The Spiritual Distress Assessment tool below highlights the prevalence and nature of Spiritual Distress among palliative care patients in India. The tool is adapted to address a different population of patients, antepartum patients. The chaplain residents and the project director indicated their responses after providing spiritual support to patients. The project director and chaplain residents dialogued about these possible responses in the attempt to spiritual distress in patients.

1. The patient is angry because of what is happening to them.

2. The patient feels that God is with them.

3. The patient feels that since the onset of their illness, they have become less interested in thinking about God and religion.

---

135 Joris Gielen, Sushma Bhatnagar, Santhosh K. Chaturvedi; Prevalence and Nature of Spiritual Distress Among Palliative Care Patients in India. Journal of Religion and Health (2017) 56: 530-544.

4. The patient wonders what will happen after . . . [the event].

5. God is a source of peace for the patient.

6. The patient is afraid of the future.

7. Thinking about what will happen after . . . [the event], frightens the patient.

8. The patient has a belief in God that strengthens them.

9. Patient feels abandoned by God.

10. The patient feels that with this illness, God wants to punish them.

In addition to the Spiritual Assessment Tool, I read and provided feedback to chaplain residents based on the focus notes that they wrote in electronic logging. The chaplain reviewed the notes and provided one-on-one helpful feed-back to the chaplain residents who wrote about their dialogues with patients. The better part of this exercise was initiated in the class sessions when residents had just completed their visitations with patients. The Spiritual Assessment Tool was to introduce and provide an opportunity to dialogue about chaplain residents' comfort levels in providing pastoral support to antepartum patients. The other pastoral skills in the spiritual assessment tool were to learn ways to assess the basic fears or spiritual distress from the patient's perspective. Most of the chaplain residents' focus notes reflected good dialogues with patients. Most of the cases were discussed openly in class.

I explained to chaplain residents the importance of working on improved listening skills with patients. This was especially challenging for one chaplain resident who felt uncomfortable on her visit. The chaplain resident noted in class how difficult it was for her to listen to the graphic details about the patient's medical condition as well as details about her personal life. Her focus note did not include the descriptive details of many of the patient's story. The chaplain resident discussed her discomfort about the details to me, the class facilitator. I listened and affirmed her uneasiness. I also impressed upon the resident the spiritual healing that may come from patients when they share their pain with others. The chaplain resident agreed to return to visit the same patient after the discussion. The chaplain resident took this as a challenge. At the next class session, she reported how successful her second visit went. She noted that the patient thanked her for listening to her story. The chaplain's second focus note gave fewer details than the last note but reflected her compassion and improved helping skills to the patient.

APPENDIX G

Electronic Documentations and Focus Notations

The Allscripts/Gateway Eclipsys electronic logging helps chaplains document their visits with patients. Key words and phrases point out the kind of patient, the needs of the patient, and other words to reflect what was accomplished on the visit. There are several categories that can be checked off that show how the chaplain provided support to the patient. An enclosed space for a paragraph summation by the chaplain is also provided. Such things as time, type, outcomes, and referral or consult information is available for all to see on the healthcare team. These notes can be seen in all disciplines, clinical areas and service lines across the Baylor Dallas campus. These notes are available as long as the patient is in the hospital or in the current system for the duration of their time at Baylor.

Chaplain E-logs are specific to the Office of Missions and Ministry (OMM). Chaplains can indicate significant details that contain familiar words and phrases specific to the pastoral care culture. These notes are available to the pastoral care team annually and allow for easy access for all chaplains to see on the campus. This system provides significant information for all chaplains to see. Pastoral care orders, patient requests for visits, and the general maintenance needed to document the number of times chaplains have visited the patient. These visit requests come to the OMM triage desk, where chaplains are assigned to visit a variety of patients with many needs.

The paragraph space provided in both of focus notes affords the chaplain the opportunity to detail the essence of the visit from the chaplain's perspective.

APPENDIX H

Spiritual Journey Genogram[136]

Using the diagram as an example, chaplain residents designed their personal genograms and later helped patients develop their personal genograms. Participants included in their genograms, individual church histories, key relatives, and others who inspired them in their faith journeys. Noting important dates and occasions can mark significant milestones in the patients' spiritual histories.

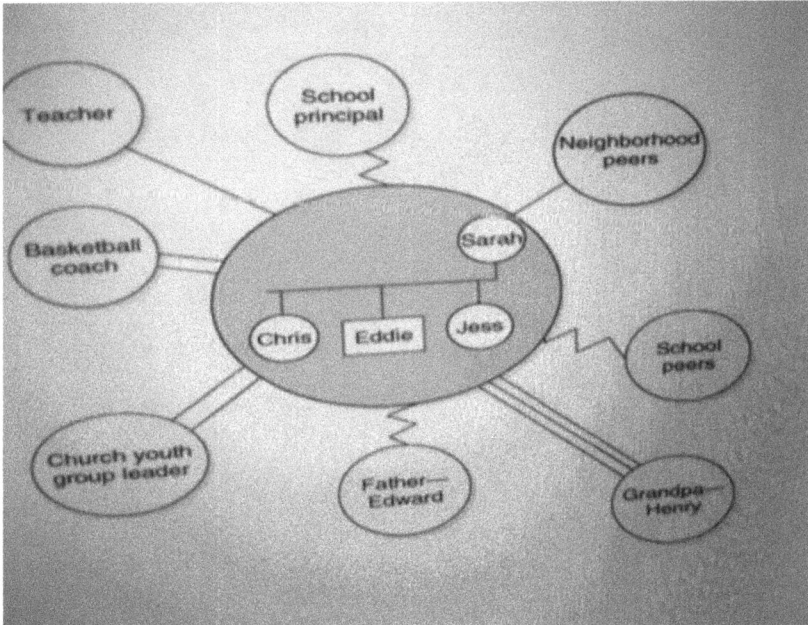

---

136 Friedman, Generation to Generation. The project director and chaplain residents completed SJG's to inform themselves about selected theological themes in Appendix 8, 97.

Bibliography

Primary Sources

Books

Cassell, Eric J. *The Nature of Suffering and the Goals of Medicine*. 2nd ed. Oxford, England: Oxford University Press, 2004.

Easley, Kendall H., and Christopher Morgan, eds. *The Community of Jesus: A Theology of the Church*. Nashville: Broadman and Holman Publishers Group, 2013.

Glasscock, Ed. Matthew. *Moody Commentary*. Chicago: Moody Press, 1997.

Habermas, Gary R. *Why is God Ignoring Me? What to Do When It Feels Like He's Giving You the Silent Treatment*. Carol Stream, IL: Tyndale House Publishers, 2010.

Herdman, T. H., and S. Kamitsuru. *Spiritual Distress 2015-2017: Definitions and Classification*. Boston: Wiley-Blackwell, 2014.

Holst, Lawrence E., ed. *Hospital Ministry: The Role of the Chaplain Today*. Eugene, OR: Wipf & Stock Publishers, 1985.

Janowsky, Bernd. *Arguing with God: A Theological Anthropology of the Psalms*. Louisville, KY: Westminster/John Knox, 2013.

Koenig, Harold G. *Spirituality and Health Research: Methods, Measurement, Statistics, and Resources*. West Conshohocken, PA: Templeton Press, 2011.

Nouwen, Henri J. M. *The Wounded Healer: In Our Own Woundedness, We Can Become a Source of Life for Others*. New York: Image Books Doubleday, 1990.

Reeves, Rodney. *Spirituality According to Paul: Imitating the Apostle*. Downers Grove, IL: IVP Academic, 2011.

Rogers, Dale Evans. *Angel Unaware*. Grand Rapids: Baker Books, 1981.

Ryrie, Charles Caldwell. *The Role of Women in the Church*. Nashville: Academic 2011.

Stone, Howard W., and Jane O. Duke. *How to Think Theologically*. 3rd ed. Minneapolis: Fortress Press, 2013.

Wilkes, C. Gene. *Jesus on Leadership: Timeless Wisdom on Servant Leadership*, Nashville: LifeWay, 1998.

ARTICLES

Berger, Thomas, ed. "Perinatal Care at the Limit of Viability between 26 Completed Weeks of Gestation in Switzerland." Swiss Medical Weekly 10, no. 4414 (October 18, 2011): 1-3.

Carr, Simonetta. "John Knox Pastor and Prophet." New Horizons in the Orthodox Presbyterian Church 35, no. 9 (October 2014): 3-4.

Fout, Jason, A. "What Do I Fear When I Fear My God? A Theological Re-examination of a Biblical Theme." *Journal of Theological Interpretation 1, no. 9* (Spring 2015): 23.

Janowski, Bernd. "Arguing with God: A Theological Anthropology of the Psalms." *Theology Today 71*, no. 3 (2014): 352-65.

Kurth, Elisabeth. "Crying Babies, Tired Mothers: Challenges of the Post-Natal Hospital Stay: An Interpretive Phenomenological Study." *Pregnancy and Childbirth* (2010): 1-10.

McGiffert, Townley Barnes. "Children's Chaplain." *Journal of Pastoral Care and Counseling* (Summer 2002): 196.

_____. "Pastoral Counseling as a Spiritual Practice: An Exercise in a Theology of Spirituality." *Journal of Pastoral Care and Counseling 56*, no. 2 (Summer 2002): 105-212.

Snodgrass, Jill L. "A Psycho-Spiritual Family-Centered Theory of Care for Mothers in the NICU." *Journal of Pastoral Care and Counseling* (March/June 2012): 1, 8.

Weaver, Doug. "Baptists and Holiness in the Nineteenth Century: A Story Rarely Told." *Wesleyan Theological Journal 49*, no. 1 (Spring 2014): 156-74.

Witsen, Scott. "What Do I Fear When I Fear My God? A Theological Re-examination of a Biblical Theme." *Journal of Theological Interpretation 9*, no. 1 (2015): 23-38.

Secondary Sources

Books

Alcorn, Randy. *The Goodness of God: Assurance of Purpose in the Midst of Suffering*. Colorado Springs: Multnomah Books, 2010.

Appleby, David W., and George Ohlschlager, eds. Transformative Encounters: *The Intervention of God in Christian Counseling and Pastoral Care*. Downers Grove, IL: InterVarsity Press, 2013.

Bloom, Benjamin S., ed. Taxonomy of Educational Objectives: The Classification of Educational Goals. New York: David McKay Co., 1956.

Butler, Trent C., ed. *Holman Bible Dictionary*. Nashville: Holman Bible Publishers, 1991.

Casiday, Augustine, ed. Constantine to C. 600. *Cambridge History of Christianity. Vol. 2. Cambridge*: Cambridge University Press, 2007.

Chafee, John, *Thinking Critically*. 8th ed. Boston: Houghton Mifflin, Co. 2006.

Collins, Francis S. *The Language of Life: DNA and the Revolution in Personalized Medicine*. New York: HarperCollins Publishers, 2010.

Cook, David. *The Moral Maze: A Way of Exploring Christian Ethics*. London: SPCK, 1983.

Dockery, David S., Gen. Ed., *Holman Bible Handbook*. Nashville: Holman Bible Publishers, 1992,

Driscoll, Mark, and Gerry Breshears. Vintage Church: *Timeless Truths and Timely Methods*. Wheaton, IL: Crossway Books, 2008.

Ferguson, Sinclair, and David Wright, eds. *New Dictionary of Theology*. Downers Grove, IL: InterVarsity Press, 1988.

Fernando, Ajith, ed. Acts. *NIV Application Commentary*. Grand Rapids: Zondervan Publishing House, 1998.

Friedman, Edwin. *Generation to Generation: Family Process in Church and Synagogue*. Guilford Family Therapy Series. 1st ed. New York: Guilford Press, 2011.

Garret, James Leo, Jr. *Systematic Theology Biblical, Historical, and Evangelical*. Vol. 1. 2nd ed. Eugene, OR: WIPF & Stock, 1990.

_____. *Systematic Theology Biblical, Historical, and Evangelical*. Vol. 1. 4th ed. Eugene, OR: WIPF & Stock, 1990.

The Grandmother's Bible: (Large Print 2010). The Holy Bible: New International Version. Grand Rapids: Zondervan Publishing House, 1984.

Gronlund, Norman E. *Measurement and Evaluation in Teaching*. New York: Macmillan Co., 1967.

Hamilton, James M. *What is Biblical Theology: A Guide to the Bible's Story, Symbolism and Patterns*. Wheaton, IL: Crossway Books, 2014.

Hays, Richard. *The Moral Vision of the New Testament: A Contemporary Introduction to New Testament Ethics*. New York: HarperCollins Publishers, 1996.

Hiltner, Seward. *Theological Dynamics*. Nashville: Abingdon Press, 1972.

Inbody, Tyron L. *The Many Faces of Christology*. Nashville: Abingdon Press, 2002.

Kirkwood, Neville A. *Pastoral Care in Hospitals*. Harrisburg, PA: Morehouse Publishing, 1998.

Lester, Andrew D. *The Angry Christian: A Theology of Care and Counseling*. Louisville, KY: Westminster/John Knox Press, 2003.

Mager, Robert F. *Measuring Instructional Results: How to Find Out if Your Instructional Objectives Have Been Achieved*. 3rd ed. Atlanta: CEP Press, 1997.

_____. *Preparing Instructional Objectives: A Critical Tool in the Development of Effective Instruction*. 3rd ed. Atlanta: CEP Press, 1997.

McDonald, H. Dermot. *Commentary on Colossians & Philemon*. Theta Books. Waco, TX: Word Books Publisher, 1980.

McLaren, Brian D. *Generous Orthodoxy: Why I am a Missional, Evangelical, Post/ Protestant, Liberal/Conservative. Mystical/Poetic, Biblical, Charismatic/ Contemplative, Fundamentalist/Calvinist, Anabaptist/ Anglican, Methodist, Catholic, Green, Incarnational, Depressed-Yet-Hopeful, Emergent, Unfinished Christian*. El Cajon, CA: Zondervan, 2004.

Oden, Thomas C. *Pastoral Theology: Essentials of Ministry*. San Francisco: Harper and Row, 1983.

Oswalt, John N., ed. *From Biblical Text . . . To Contemporary Life, Isaiah*. NIV Commentary. Grand Rapids: Zondervan, 2003.

Parker, Gary. *Creation Facts of Life: How Religion and Spiritual Health Reveals the Hand of God*. Green Forest, AR: Master Books, 2006.

Piper, John, Justin Taylor, and Paul Kjoss Helseth, eds. *Beyond the Bounds: Open Theism and the Undermining of Biblical Christianity*. Wheaton, IL: Crossway Books, 2003.

Rohrer, David. *The Sacred Wilderness of Pastoral Ministry: Preparing a People for the Presence of the Lord*. Downers Grove, IL: InterVarsity Press, 2012.

Seamands, Stephan. *Ministry in the Image of God: The Trinitarian Shape of Service*. Downers Grove, IL: InterVarsity Press, 2005.

Switzer, David K. *Pastoral Care Emergencies. Creative Pastoral Care and Counseling Series*. Minneapolis: Fortress Press, 2000.

Warren, Rick. *The Purpose Driven Church: Growth without Compromising Your Message and Mission*. Grand Rapids: Zondervan Publishing House, 1995.

Taylor, Elizabeth Johnston. "Spiritual Care: Evangelism at the Bedside?." *Journal of Christian Nursing* 28, no. 4 (2011): 194-202.

Doctoral Dissertations

Ashlock, Larry C. "Equipping Christians to Deal Effectively with the Problem of Evil and Suffering." D.Min. proj., Southwestern Baptist Theological Seminary, 1985.

Graham, Patricia E. Mahon. "Nursing Students' Perception of How Prepared They Are to Assess Patients' Spiritual Needs." Ph.D. diss., Graduate Program at the College of Saint Mary, 2008.

Hays, Cindy S. "Reclaiming the Spiritual Leadership Role of Christian Parents in Family Life: Coaching and Markers." Ph.D. diss., Liberty University Baptist Theological Seminary, 2014.

Schmidt, Angela E. "Partnerships Between Hospitals and Community: A Qualitative Study on Collaborations for Spiritual Care in Healthcare." D.Min. diss., Wilfrid Laurier University, 2013.

Electronic Sources

Gateway/Allscripts and Eclipsys Documentation IT Process [used at Baylor Scott and

White Health]. wwwhealthitnews.com/news/Allscripts-Eclipsys-match [accessed November 30, 2017].

LaRocca Pitts, Mark. "Fact: Taking a Spiritual History in a Clinical Setting." Journal of

Healthcare Chaplaincy 15, no. 1 (March 17, 2009): 1-12. www.tandfonline.
   com/doi/abs/10.1080/08854720802698350 [accessed November
   30, 2017].

_____. "Four FACT Spiritual History Tool." Journal of Healthcare
   Chaplaincy 21, no. 2 (March 20, 2015): 51-59. https://www.ncbi.nlm.
   nih.gov/pubmed/25793421 [accessed November 30, 2017].

Lippincott Nursing Center. (July 14, 2013). http://
   nursinginterventionsrationales.blog spot.com/2013/07/spiritual-
   distress.html-Minggu [accessed October 30, 2015].

Nasreen, Hashema E., Zarina N. Kabir, Yvonne Forsell, and Maigun
   Edhborg, eds. "Low Birth Weight of Off-spring with Depressive and
   Anxiety Symptoms During Pregnancy: Results from a Population
   Based Study in Bangladesh." BMC Public Health 10 (2010): 515.
   http://www.biomedcentral.com/1471 [accessed October 15, 2015].

Nursing Care Plan. "Spiritual Distress." http://wps.prenhall.
   com/wps/media/objects/3918/ 4012970/NursingTools/
   ch41NCPSpiritualDistress1055.pdf [accessed October 30, 2015].

Spiritual Distress. "Plans, Outcomes, and Interventions" (March 10,
   2007). http://www.rn central.com/nursing-library/careplans/sd-
   (NANDA) [accessed October 25, 2015].

Photos

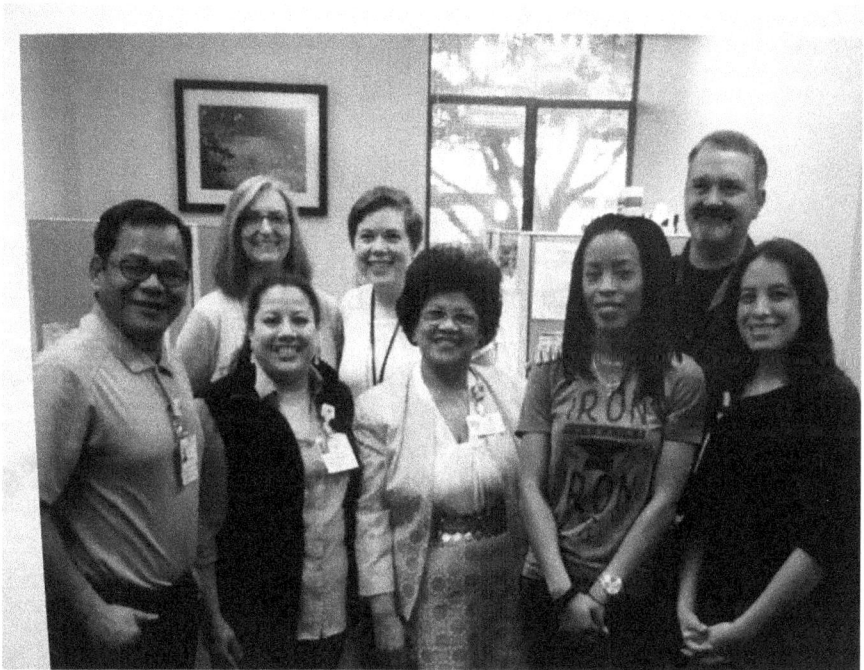

Chaplain Residents at Baylor University Medical Center Dallas, TX

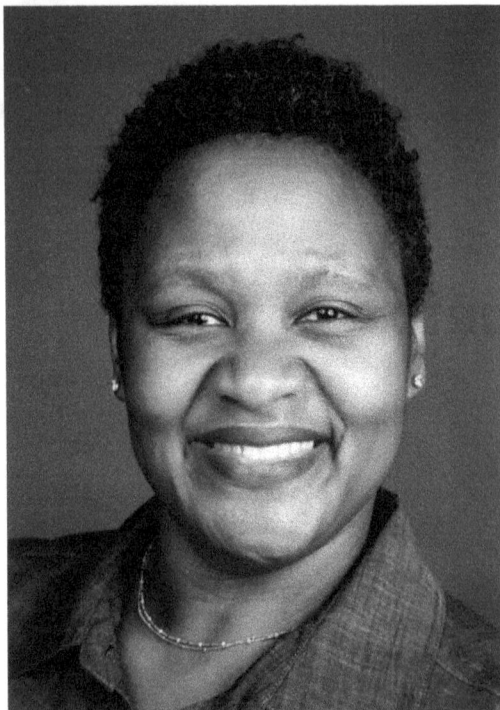

Lauren Frazier McGuin is the CPE Manager for the Office of Mission and Ministry. She offered her Theological Reflection class timeslot for my doctoral project. She also became a student of sorts which made the students comfortable with a challenging list of requirements I had for each class session. Her gentility and encouragement helped our work appear seamless.

Ella McCarroll was one of my first Clinical Coordinators when I was a summer intern in the CPE program. I learned much about the skill and care needed for Maternal Child Health patients. The introduction would be powerful when I became a staff chaplain. I was initially inspired by her class at a church convention on "grief." She empowered me.

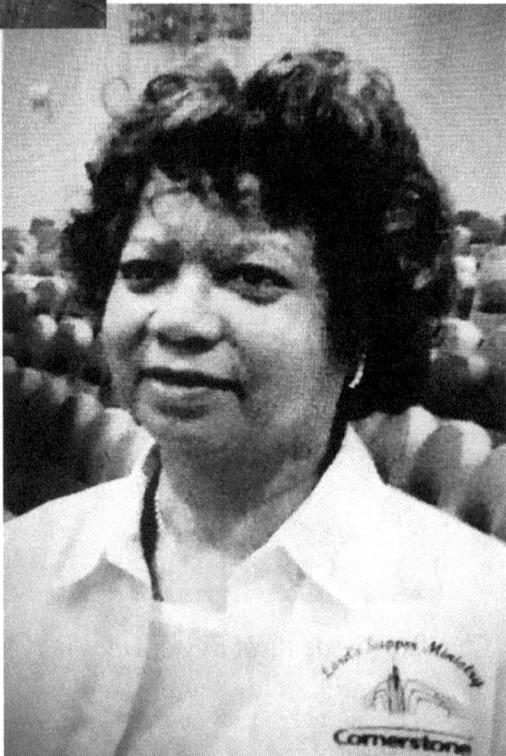

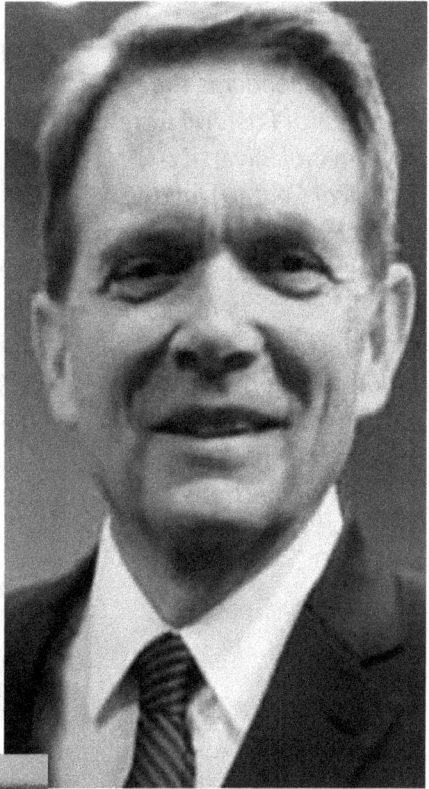

Larry Ashlock was the Dean of the Doctor of Ministry program at B.H. Carroll Institute in Irving, TX. He and Margaret Lawson guided me through the program with patience and tenacity. Their credentials are cited early in this book. I received a grant from Dr. Ashlock's non-profit organization (Baptist Center for Global Concerns) during my last semester at Carroll.

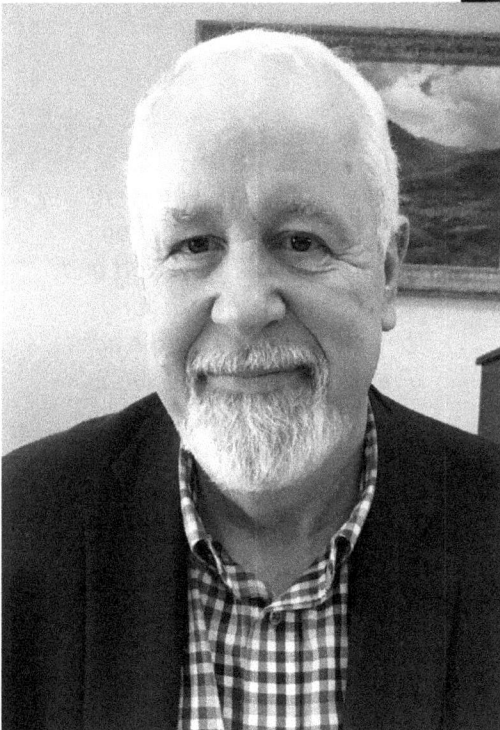

Mark Grace is the Chief Mission and Ministry Officer for all of Texas's Baylor Scott and White Health facilities and beyond. He helped me during my episode with Cancer. I am grateful that he prayed with me often, an important time of healing for me. He was an accessible servant leader who often spoke with refreshing candor

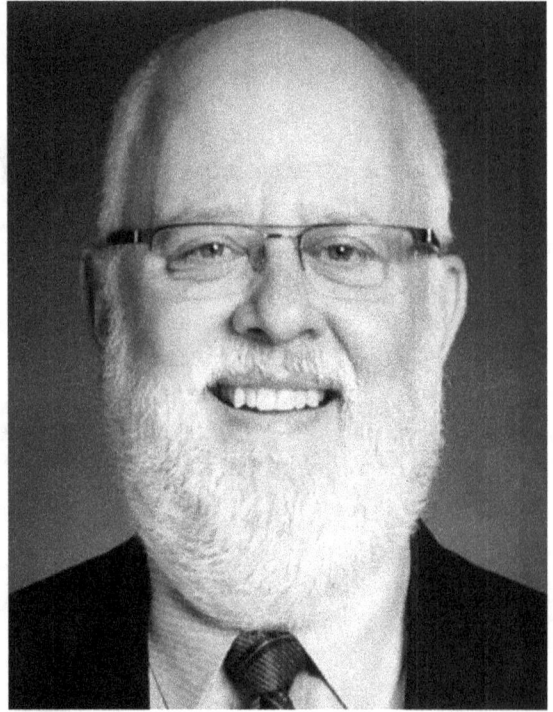

Mike Mullender is the Director of Pastoral Care for Baylor University Medical Center, Dallas Area Hospitals. He was accessible and listened always to my personal and health concerns. He asked good questions. He also sat on my doctoral project committee, providing helpful suggestions.

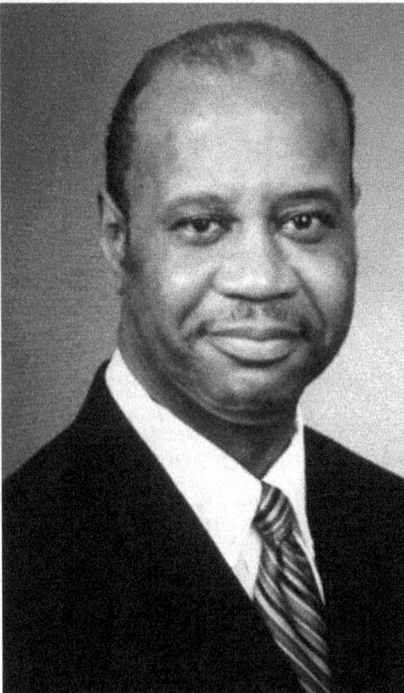

Carlos Bell is the Director of Clinical Pastoral Education Programs for Baylor Scott and White Health in Texas and beyond. He was also the past President of the Association of Clinical Pastoral Education. His listening, attending skills, and humor down the years has helped me face my fears as a woman of God.

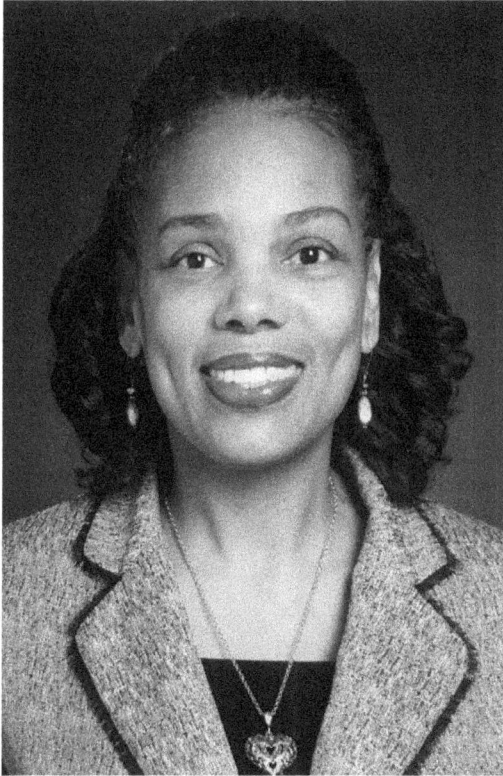

Millicent Albert is a Pastoral Care Manager. I was ecstatic when she offered me the position of Chaplain Fellow and later as Staff Chaplain. Her humility yet strong servant leadership empowered me as she listened to my concerns throughout difficult patient visitations. I grew to appreciate her wisdom as I approached the needs of all labor and delivery patients.

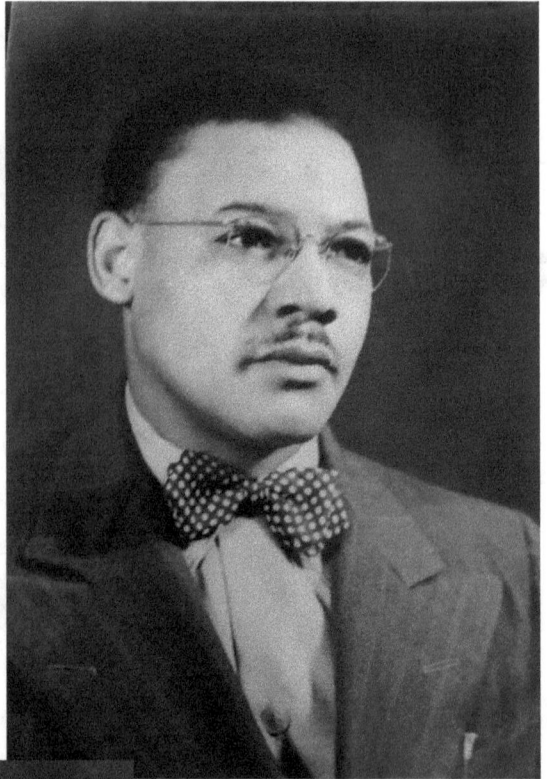

My Father John Sumner Barge (Posthumously-p) Strong, loving disciplinarian who inspired us in academia. Died in his 50's. He was a letter carrier for the downtown Norfolk business district. Excellent provider for his family.

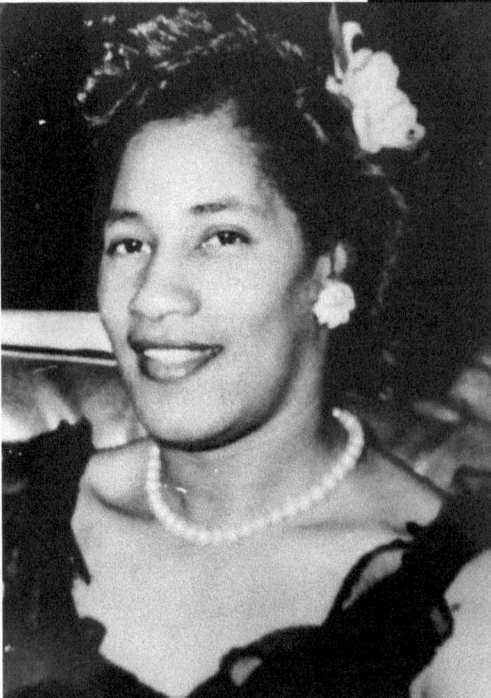

My Mother Willie Langley Barge-p Superb household organizer. Stanley Home Product Saleswoman. A diligent mother whose wise sayings and actions modeled the beauty and strength of womanhood for me. She later was licensed by the city of Norfolk for home daycare.

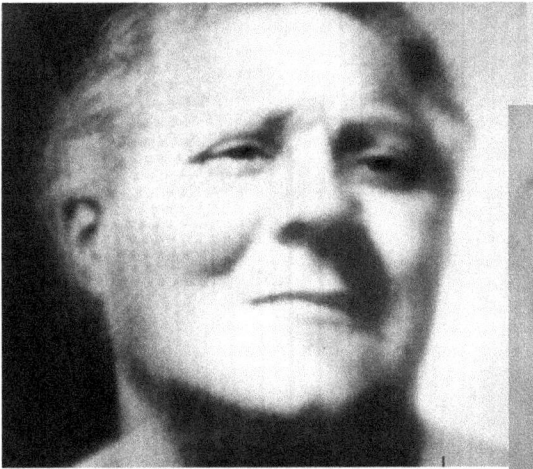

ABOVE: Lucretia Ann Sumner-p
Paternal Great Grandmother

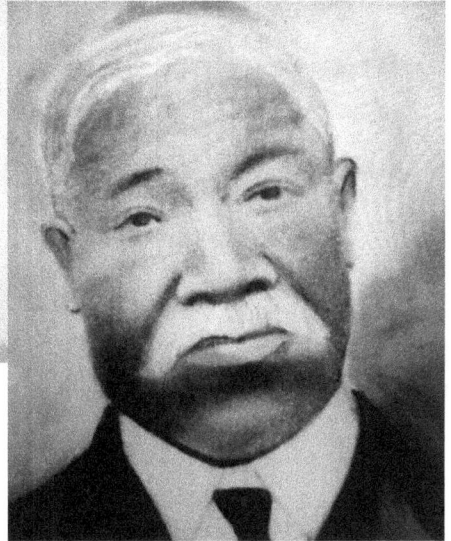

RIGHT:Mills Sumner Paternal Great
Grandfather-p

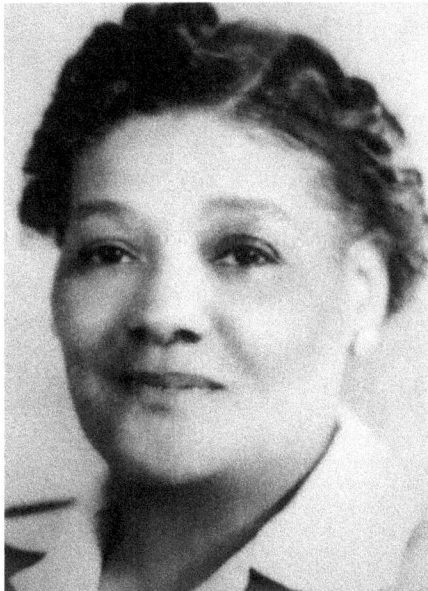

LEFT: My paternal grandmother, Adele Sumner Barge-p. Strong and
witty, always challenging her grandchildren with memorable sayings.
RIGHT: Cicero Barge-p, our paternal grandfather. I never met him. He
died the year I was born. He was in the navy. I would like to have met
him.

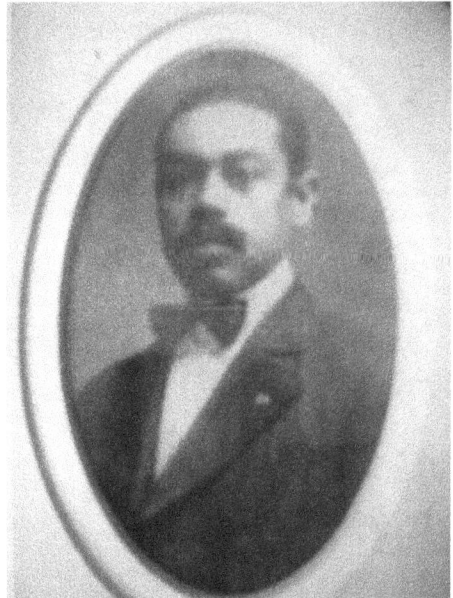

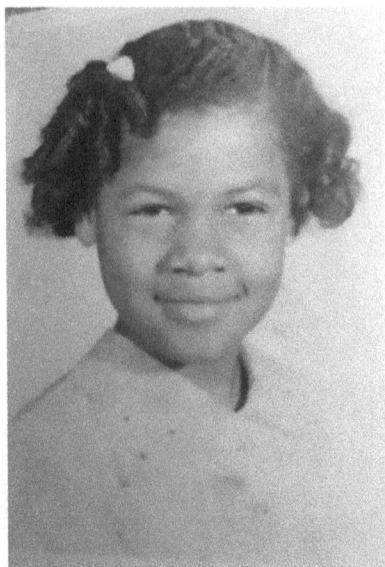

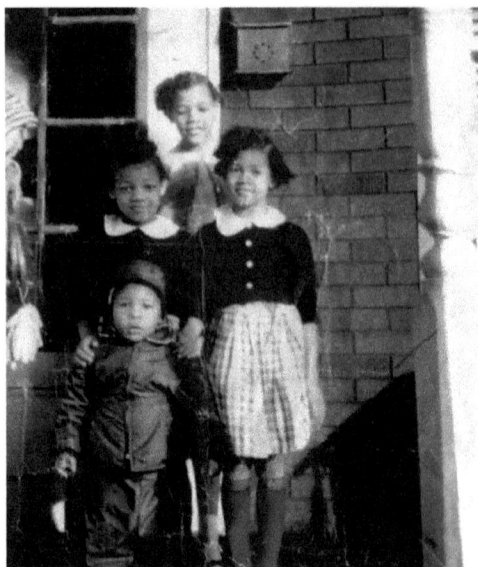

TOP LEFT: Me Age Six Liberty Park Elementary School- First Grade

TOP RIGHT: The Homestead on Anne Street. Sisters Eve and Jessie-p & Nephew Luther visiting-p

BELOW: Sixth Grade Graduation Lott Carey Elementary School/ Me- First Row-Right Center

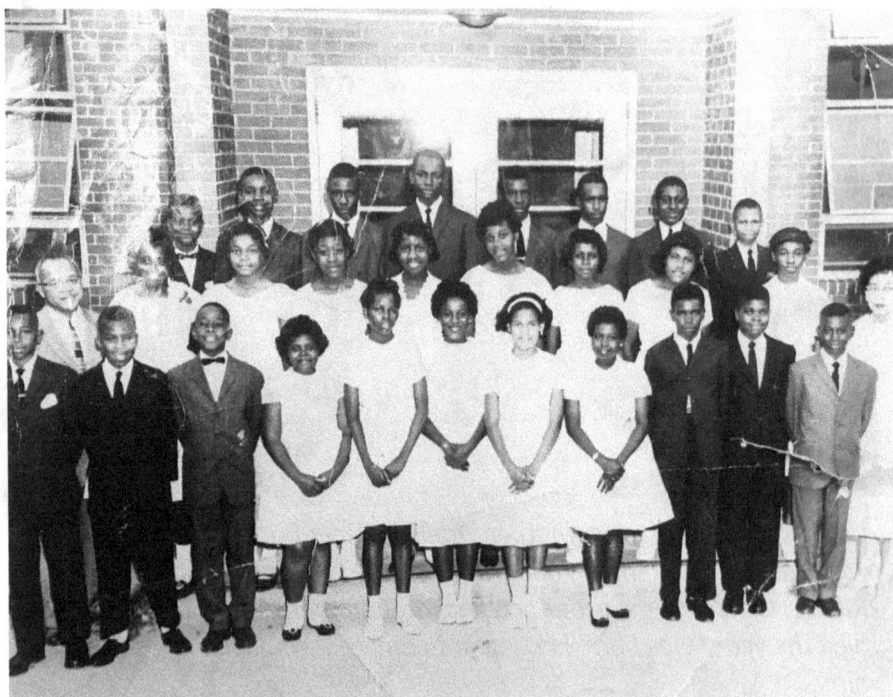

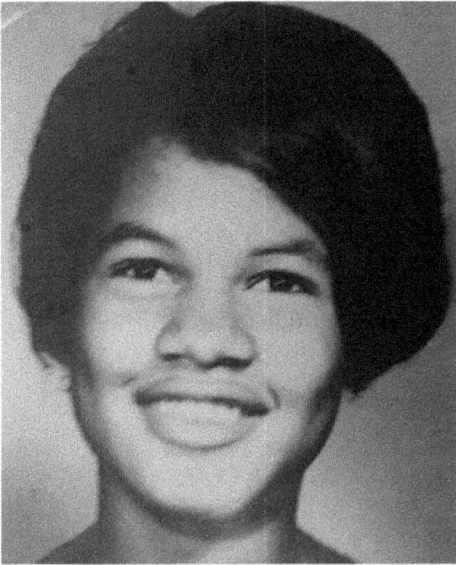

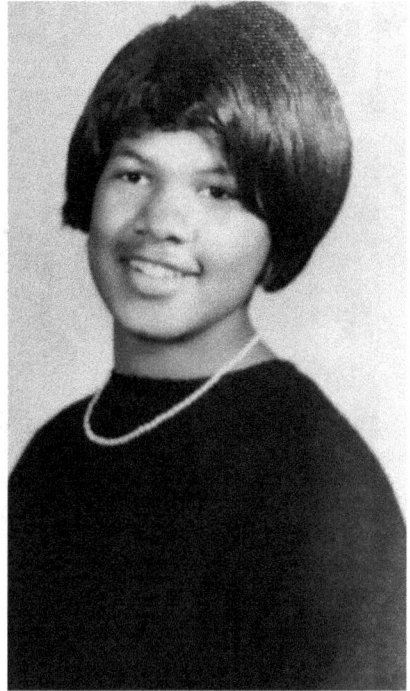

ABOVE: Jacox Junior High School
Norfolk, VA

RIGHT: Senior High School Booker T.
Washington Norfolk, VA

BELOW:Our Home on Covenant
Street Norfolk, VA

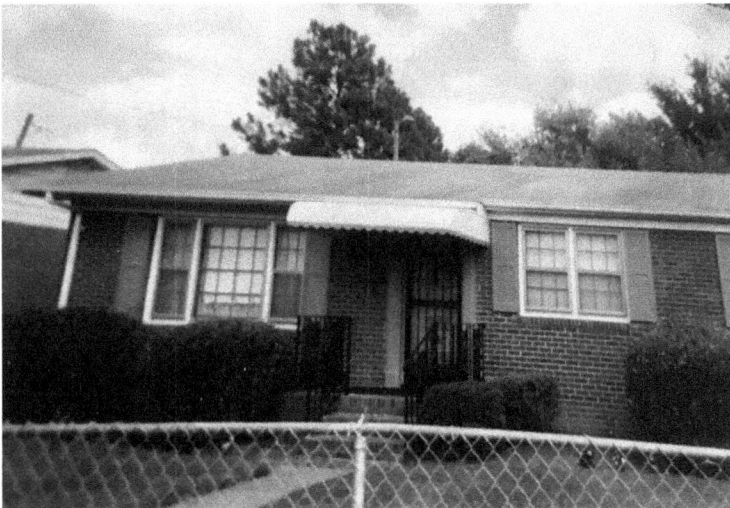

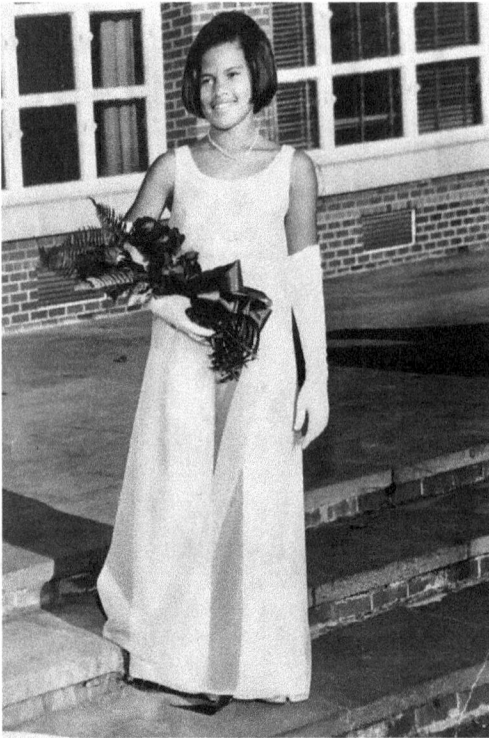

LEFT: High School Debutante Bachelor Benedict Club Norfolk State College (Now University)

BELOW: Summer Camp Counselor Arts & Crafts Camp Eleanor Young Chesapeake, VA

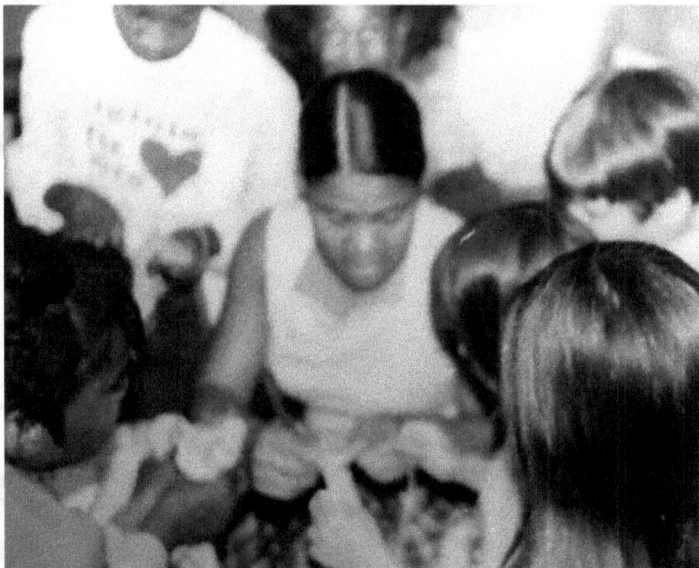

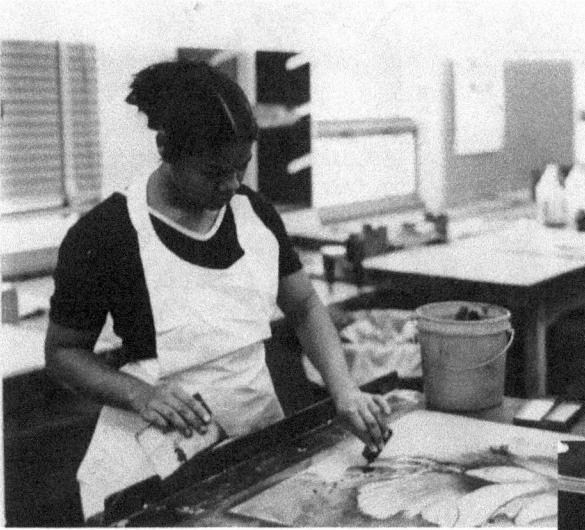

ABOVE: VA Commonwealth University Preparing a Lithograph Series

RIGHT: VA Commonwealth University Art Education. I went on a pilgrimage to Israel and Rome during my teaching years.

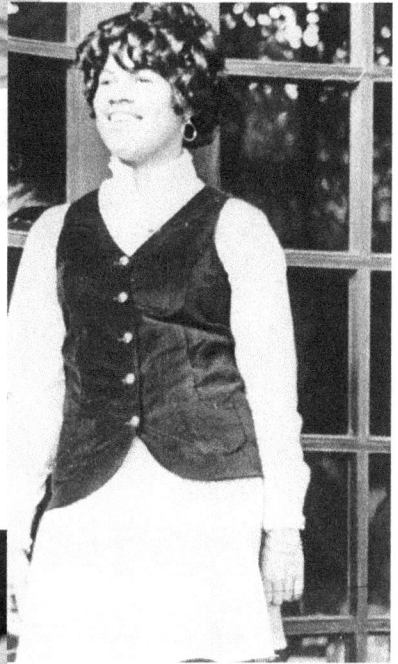

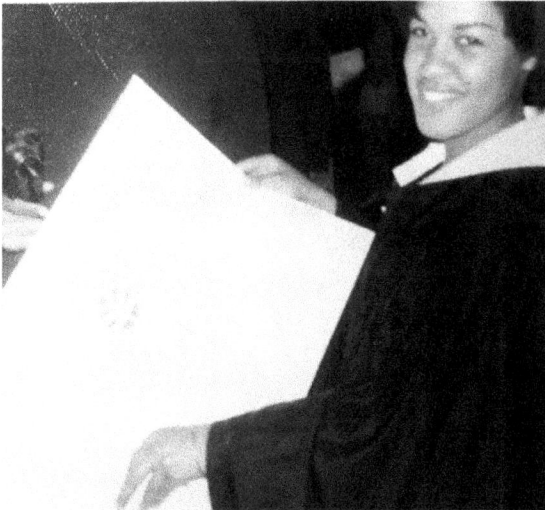

LEFT: VA Commonwealth University Graduation Bachelor of Fine Arts in Art Education

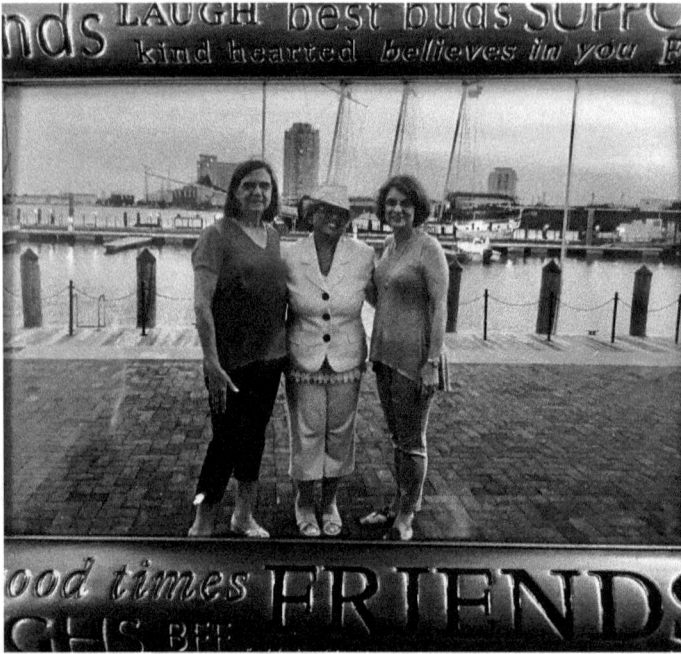

LEFT: Lasting Friendships - Dormitory College Mates Maintain Family Ties Meal Celebrations

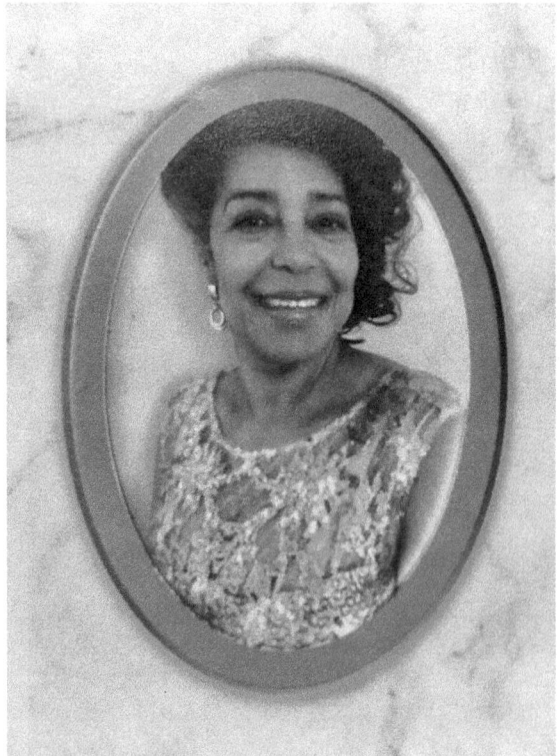

RIGHT: College Dormitory Mate, Barbara, One Inspiration for Doctorate She Completed a Doctorate Earlier

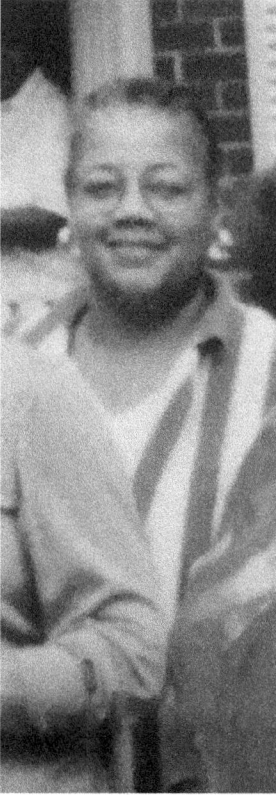

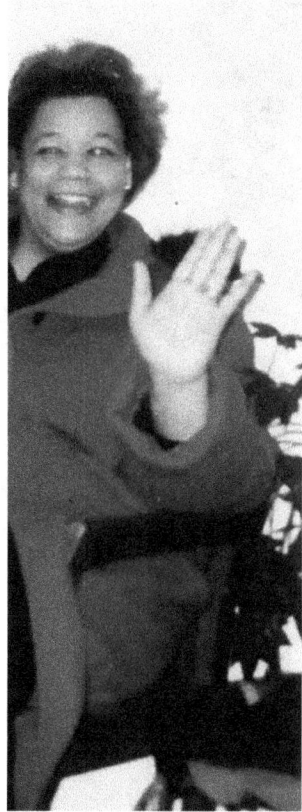

ABOVE LEFT: Jessie, our youngest sister-p, just transitioned to her eternal reward (February 2020). My constant prayer warrior. Her popular sentiment was to "Endure," just like Jesus. Her children, Sam, Esther, Mark, Ruth & Adam visited us often. From Norfolk to Richmond. We always enjoyed them with our children. We are proud of. We all miss her, she was one of my greatest confidantes.

ABOVE RIGHT: Eve is our sister, third above the youngest, the family's "resident family counselor." She asks good questions. She has had key roles in her church supporting the needs of the disenfranchised, especially women. Her creativity in church programs and in her home are well reflected in the lives of her children over the years. (Marcy (Steve-p), Alison, Dwayne (Kim), & Danielle.

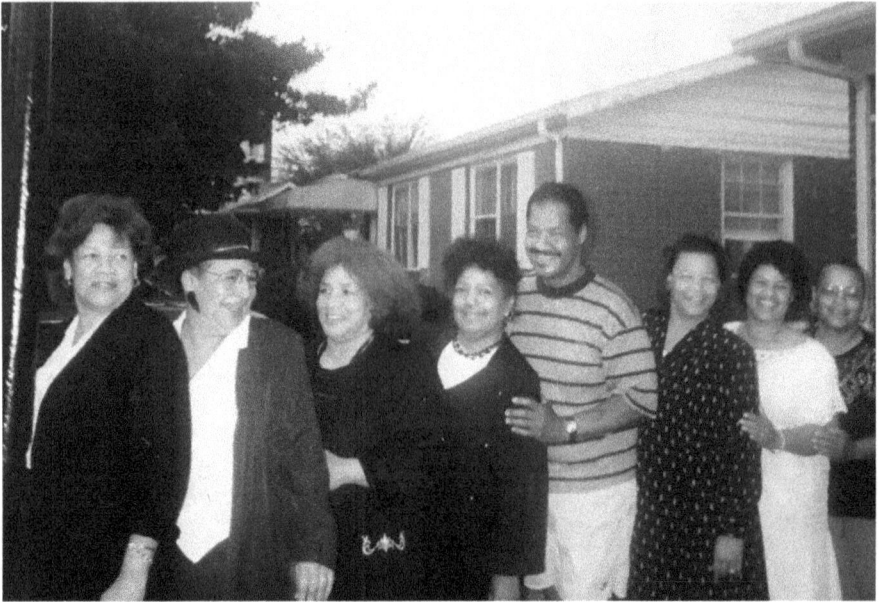

Our only brother Mike -p, (John Jr.) Minister. He loved the sport of basketball and rounded up games at family events. He had a strong sense of family and talked about practical Christian Theology often. He was an encourager.

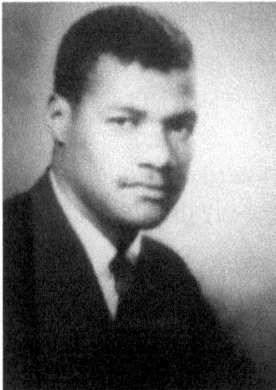

LEFT: John Barge -p, Jr

BELOW: Mike's (p) wife, (minister) Jean in California, truly our sister. She, Mike & 5 Children (John, Darby Marcus, Megan & Joy often had alternate great family vacations at our homes in TX & CA. We all bonded well.

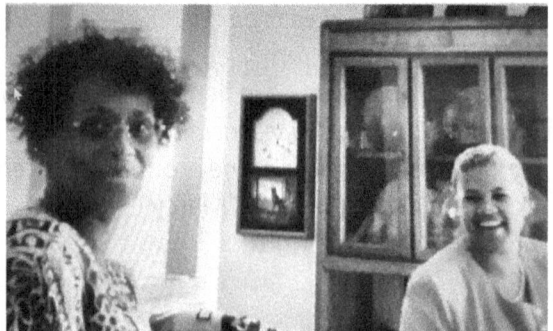

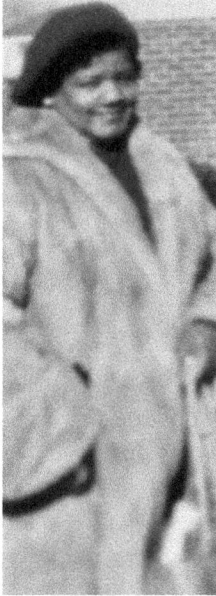

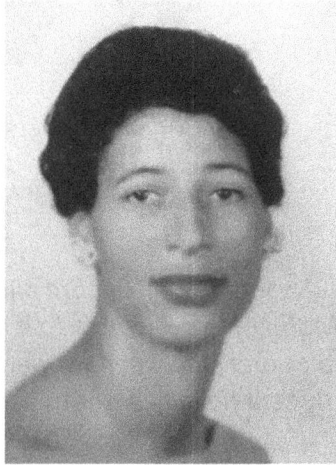

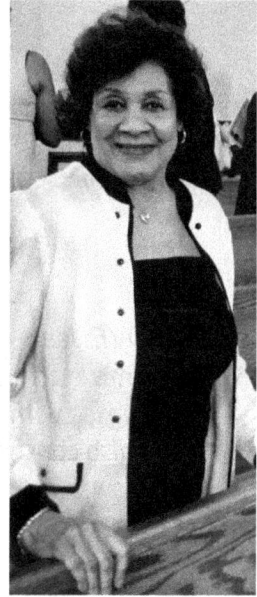

LEFT: Bernice, our 4th oldest sister is the professional woman who wisely introduced her younger sisters to the outside world. She continued to model high moral character for us. Her husband Gilbert-p and Sheldon interchanged visits to our homes in VA and MD. We are very proud of Sheldon's world-wide professional career.

CENTER: Sister Estelle. Sister who has a love for academia. She is witty and uses the humor to help others. She is a woman of faith.Her son Luther (-p) was the apple of the family's eye.

RIGHT: Jackie, the "queen." Firstborn of our parents. Our true classy & comedic "matriarch" who encourages all of her siblings to bring their "A" game. Her son Trey has acquired like qualities filled with humor and professionalism.

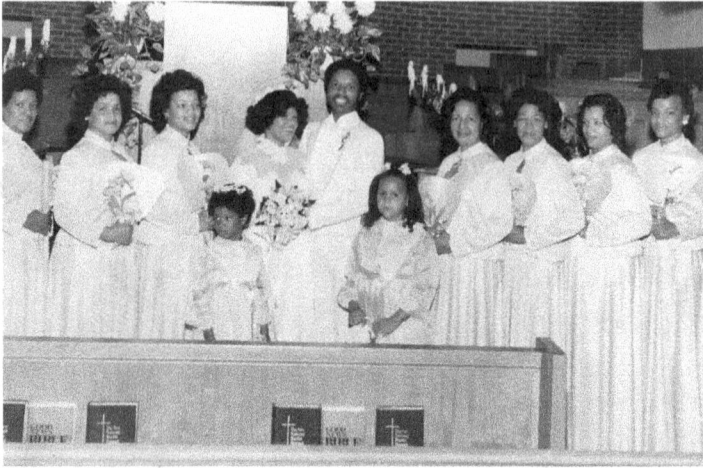

ABOVE: Jean-p, 2nd from the left. Our 3rd oldest sister, whom we called "Mother Hen." She saw to it that we had gift boxes with clothes and food when we were in college. She also consistently sent holiday boxes to her nieces and nephews.

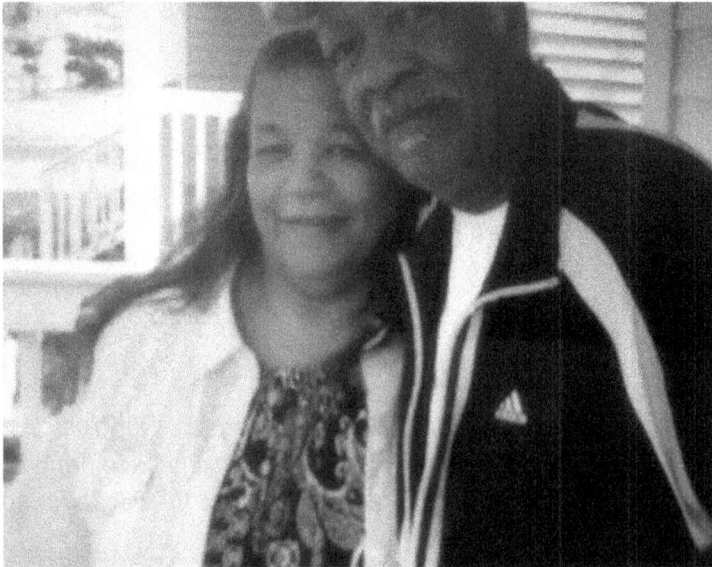

ABOVE: Eve and Bill. Classy powerful couple. Warm hospitality permeates their home. They both model compassion for others, especially the sick, in a genuine way.

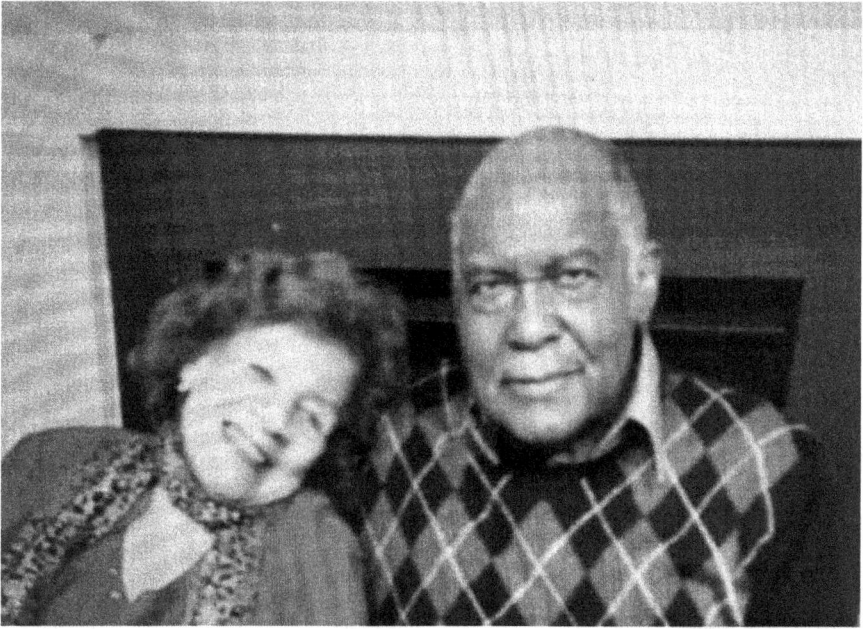

Jackie and Robert hail as the classy & suave dynamic duo everyone wants to be around. They both have a flair of excellency in service for needs within their reach. They are genuine.

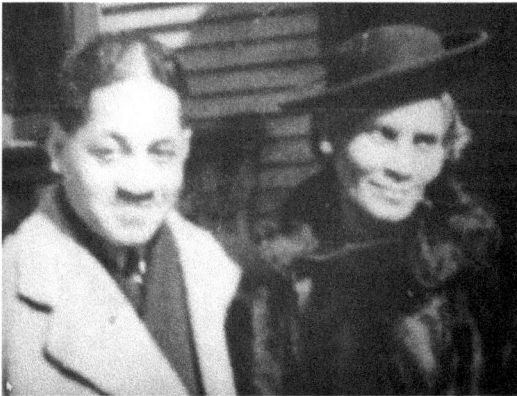

Uncle Dan and my Maternal grandmother Estelle Langley

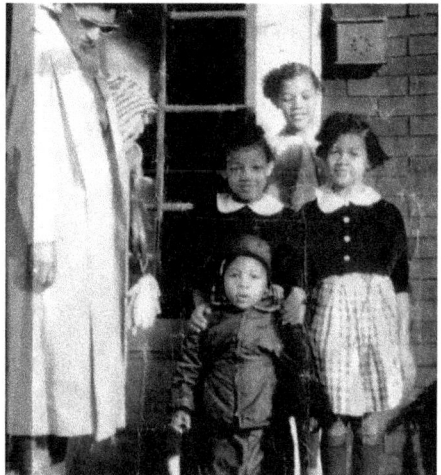

Aunt Helen-p, (Reggie-p), Jessie-p, Eve, Inez, Jessie and Luther-p, at the homestead on Anne St. in Norfolk.

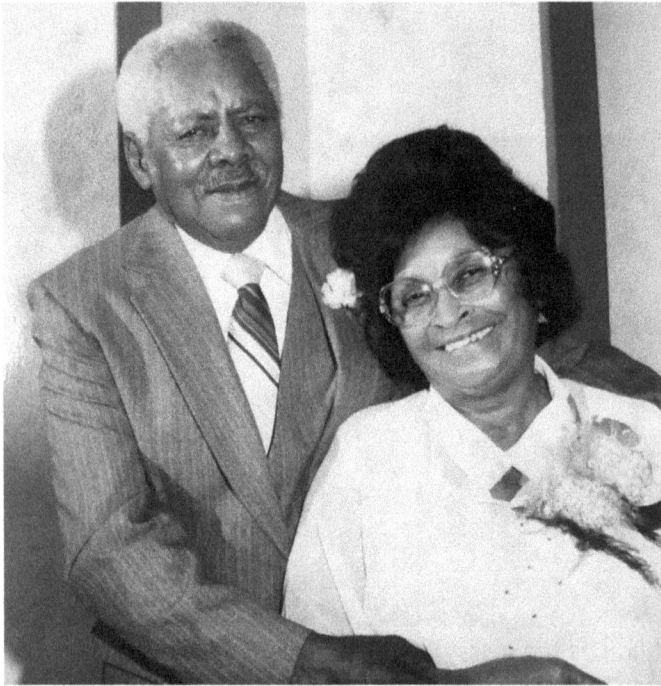

ABOVE: Husband's Parents -p
XL & Mary B. Cotton-p Father
Predicted Our Wedding and
did not live to see it. Before
Marriage, Roy's mother
came to VA to meet Inez's
Mother. They both were strong
believers in Christ.

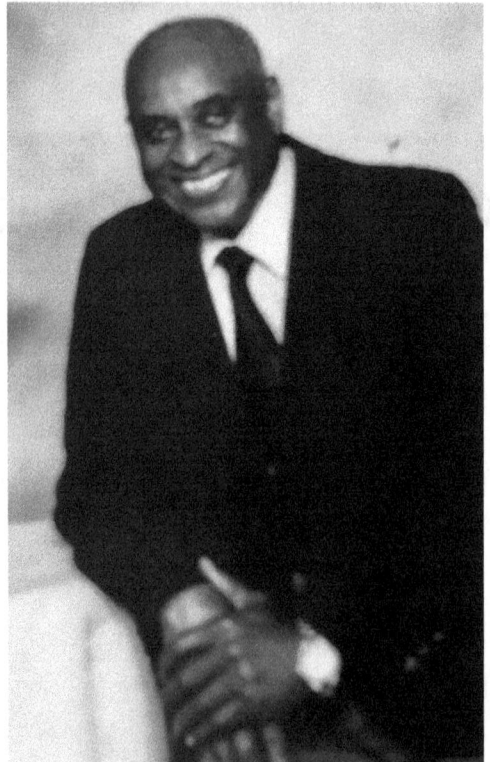

RIGHT: "XL." Brother-in-
law Donor for Entrance
Requirements & First Semester
at BH Carroll Theological
Institute, Irving, TX Family
Patriarch

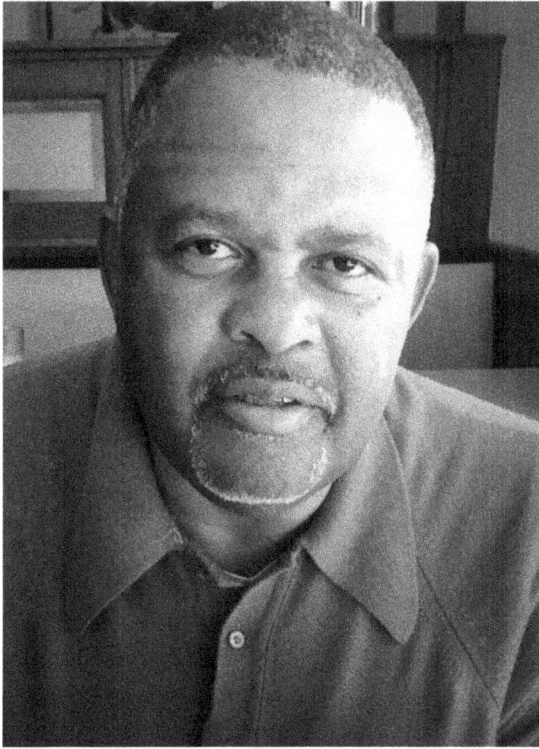

"Palmer" Brother-in-law. Compassionate Church Deacon. Has a heart for the sick. He enjoys learning about Cotton & Baxter family history.

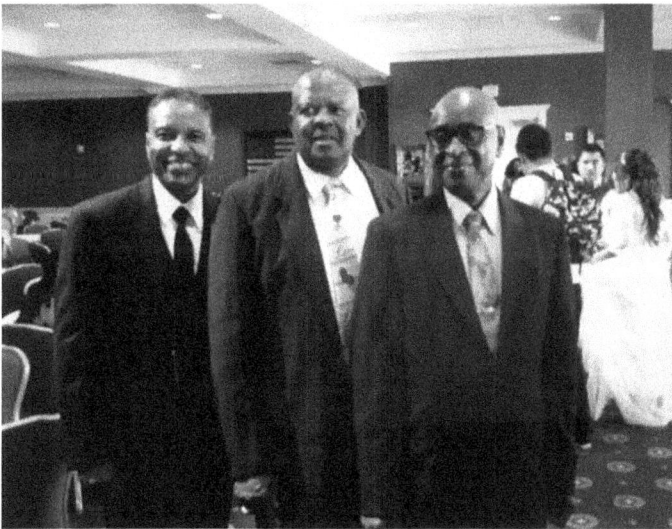

Roy, Palmer & XL Brother at Justin & Carolina's Wedding.

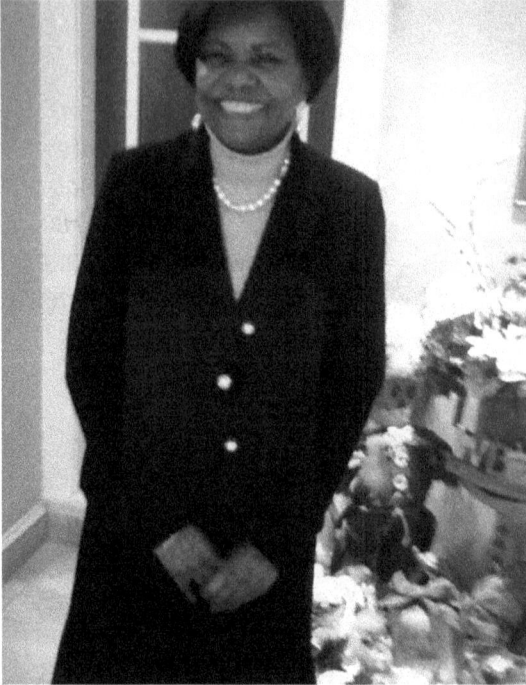

LEFT: Gwen from CA Husbands Cousin Who Shows up at Most Family Events. A Strong Family Supporter. Dynamic "super glue" for the whole family

BELOW: Cindy-p, Donna, Roy & Dorothy. Roy's Cousins from both the Maternal & Paternal sides of his family. True Texas "Sisters" to me. Beside Donna (brother Don and Cousin Adoria (Glenn) not in photo).

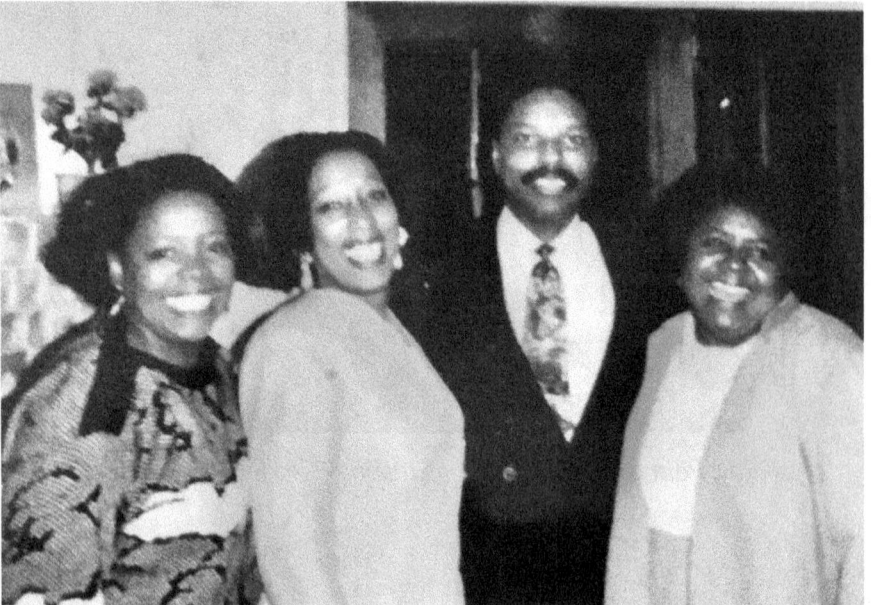

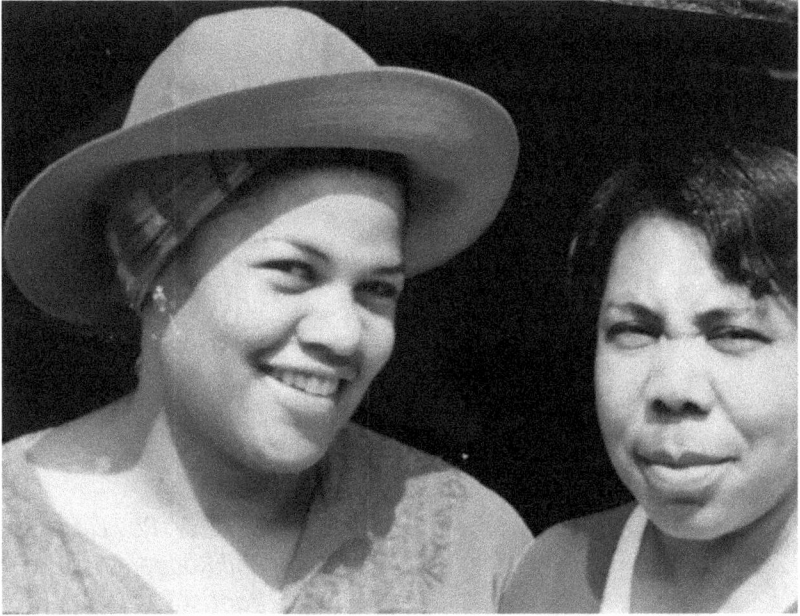

ABOVE: Joyce, Our Sister-in-law. My faithful prayer partner Palmer's wife. We dated the brothers around the same time. We enjoy godly laughter.

BELOW: Georgia-p. We Were "Girls." XL's Wife, Our Sister-in law. We Enjoyed Their Co Hospitality in Their Home in NJ.

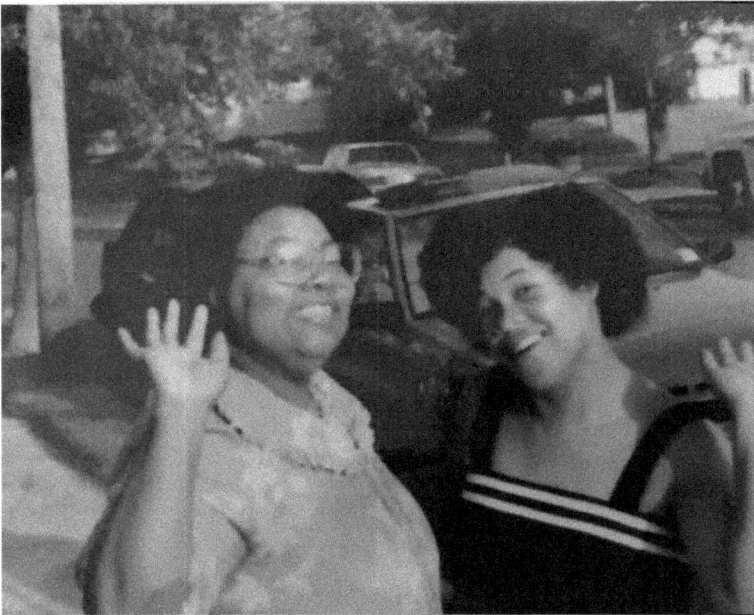

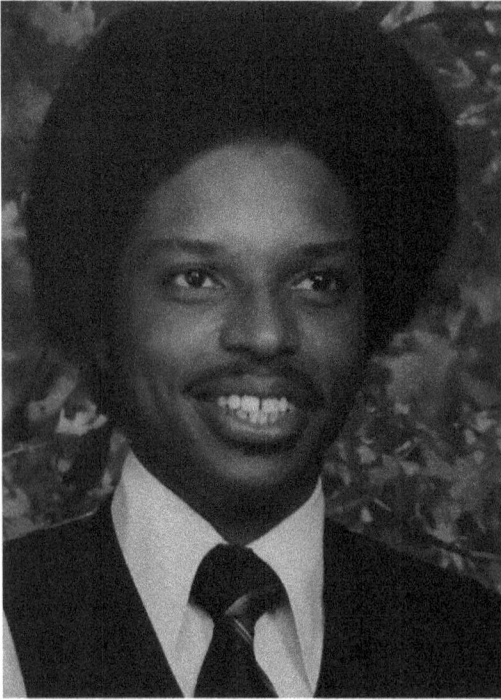

LEFT: Single Roy. Mother knew he was "the one," When my sister Jessie was seriously ill & hospitalized. He offered to take care of his nieces and nephews after marriage. He moved from Texas to Virginia and worked for Virginia Baptists.

BELOW: Roy & Co-worker Phil Rodgerson -p. Virginia Baptist Facilitator at a Church Conference. Class on Evangelism He introduced us to one another.

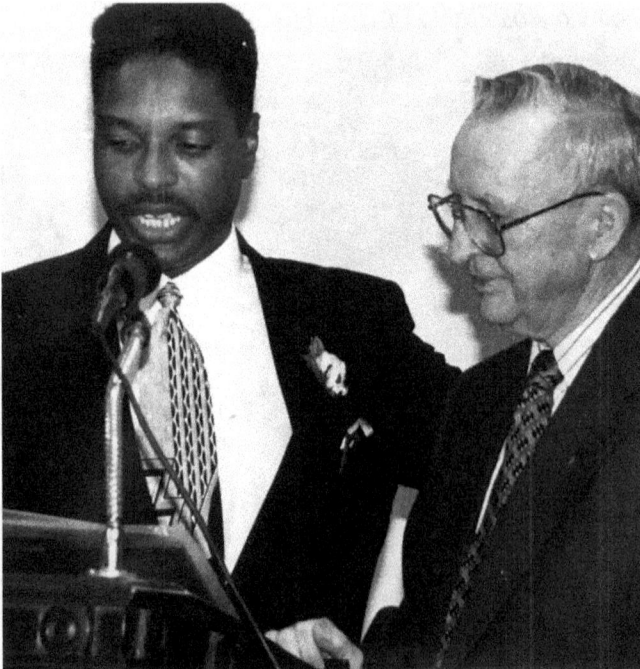

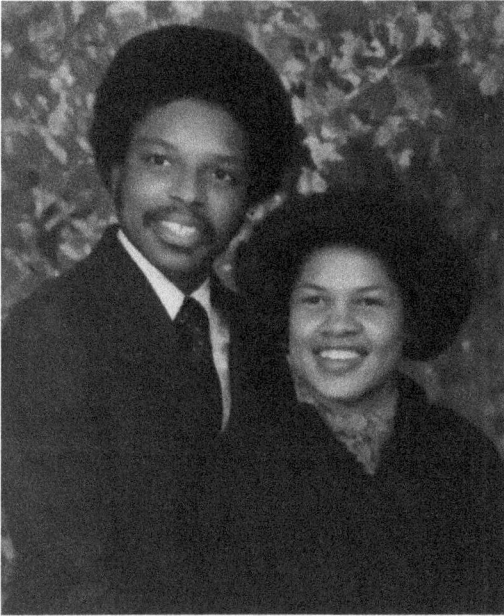

LEFT: Early Long Distance Dating Days. Roy traveled 100 miles round trip from Richmond to Norfolk. It was during these times at the Transition School, that I was introduced to many antepartum needs of high school students.

BELOW: Roy eventually meets all my six sisters. This photograph was taken in Annapolis, MD. Hollis niece far left and Mother-p far right.

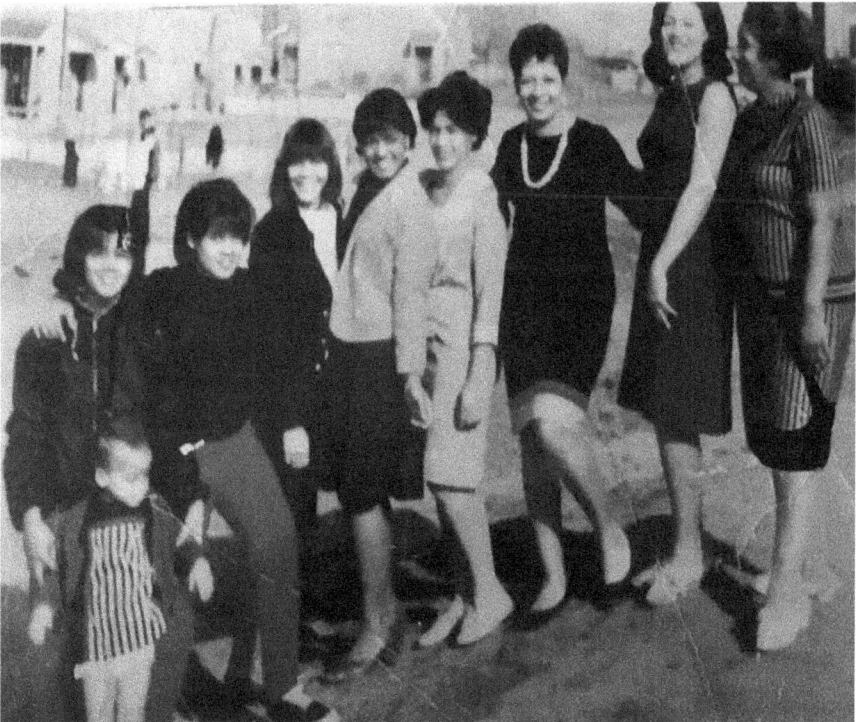

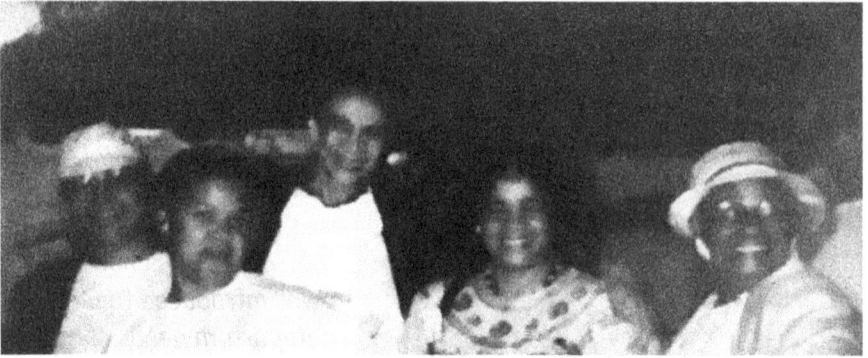

ABOVE: Adeline (center), our NY cousin. Always thoughtful with cards and good wishes. We grew up visiting her and her daughters Tina and Emily. They are great cousins; strong family ties.

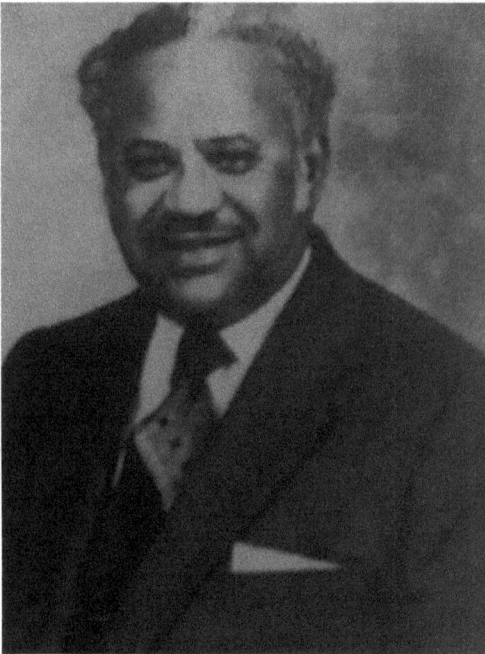

LEFT: Rev. Dr. J. B. Henderson-p (Lillian-p). Civil Rights Leader & also Supported Women in Ministry. A sound theologian, professor, and servant pastor to so many at Bank Street Memorial Baptist Church in Norfolk, VA. We admired their daughter Joyce (Aubrey), who was kind and always encouraging.

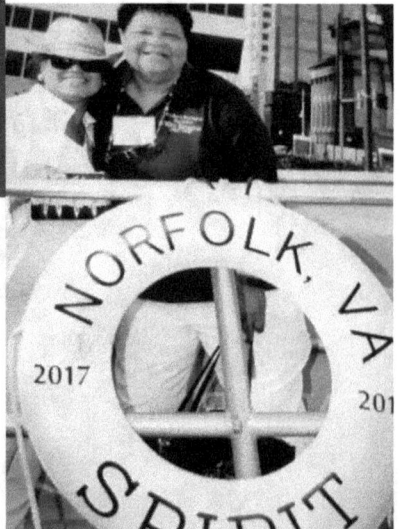

RIGHT: Mary Jane Lifetime Friendship Same Church Cruise High School Reunion

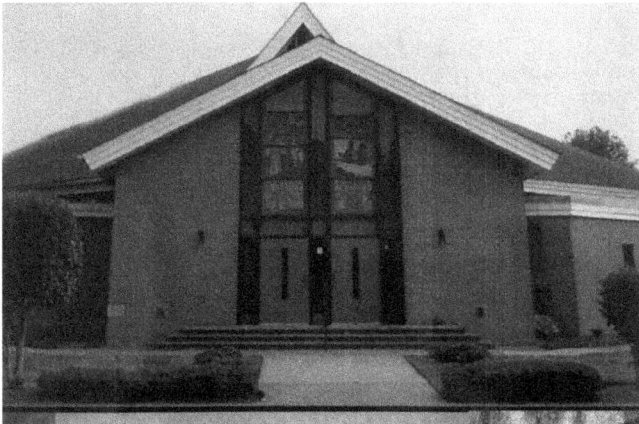

ABOVE: Bank Street Baptist Church was founded 180 years ago by freed African Americans. Roy and I were married here. To my joy, all of my sisters were bridesmaids at our wedding.

RIGHT: My newspaper engagement announcement in the Norfolk Journal & Guide, our African American newspaper.

BELOW: Rev. Dr. James C. Griffin-,p, and wife Doris-p. Retired Air Force Chaplain. (Pastor of Bank St. Church who performed our wedding). Mother invited him and wife when Roy's mother was visiting from Dallas, TX.

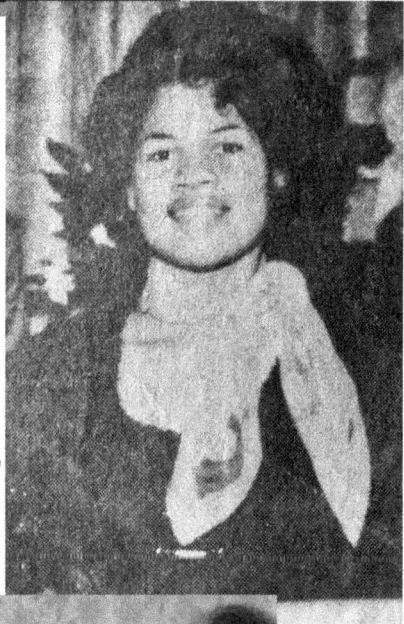

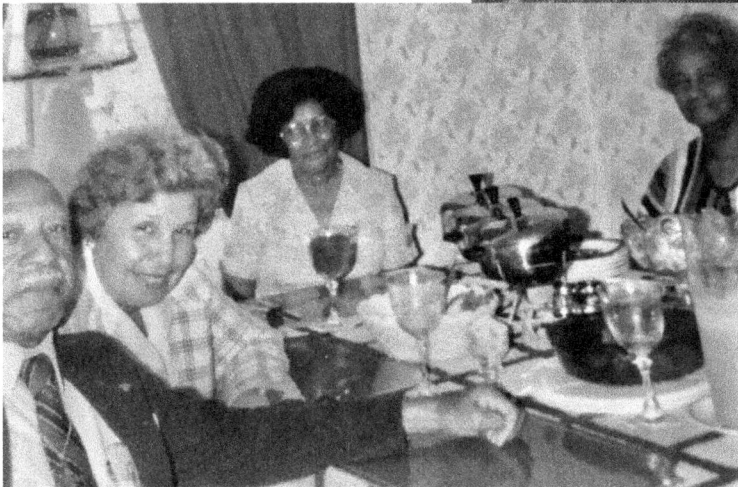

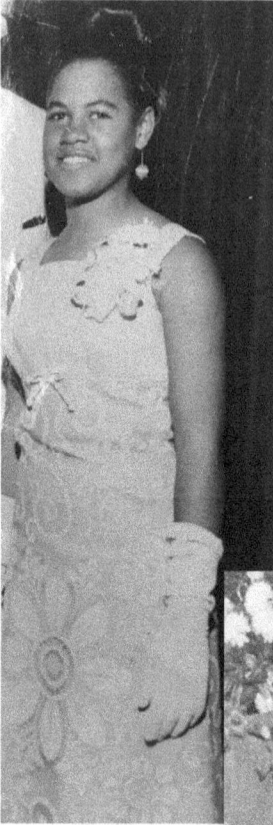

LEFT: Senior Prom High School, Class of 1967. My brother Mike bought my dress.

BELOW: Notice the candles on our wedding day. The greatest and hottest day ever. Fifth Street Baptist Church. Pastor and people came from Richmond, VA. The church was packed. Roy's family and friends traveled from NJ, TX & DC.

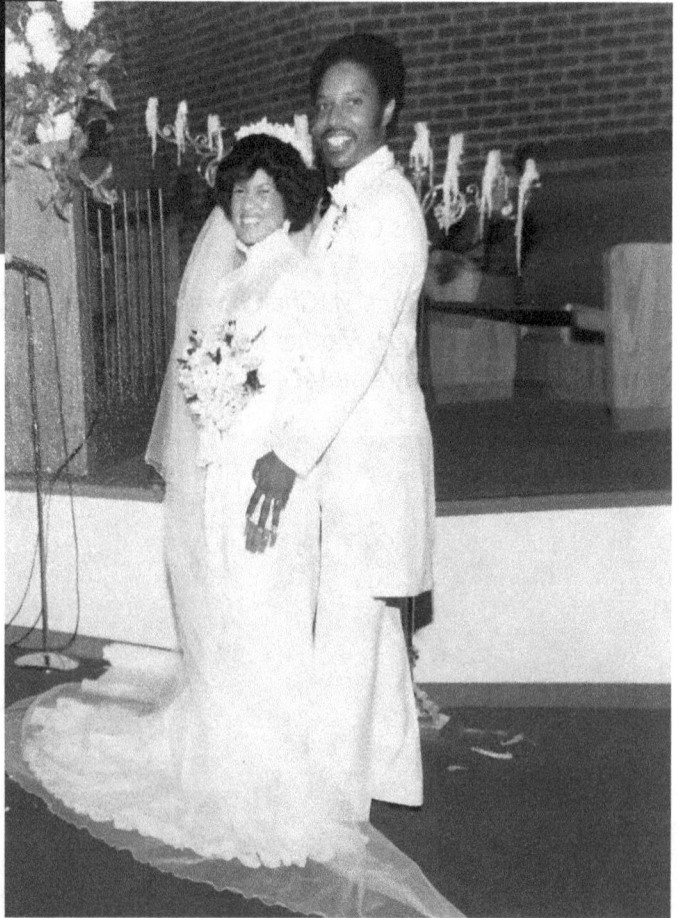

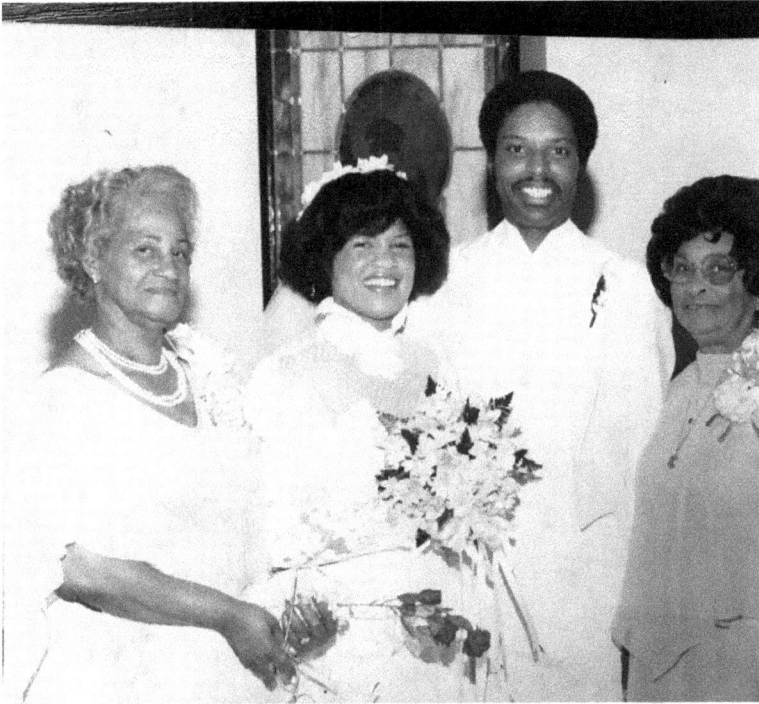

ABOVE: Wedding photograph with our mothers. Their dresses were made of the same material, to their surprise, having never talked about their choices. We were the "Last of the Mohicans," in our homes to leave the "nest." A beautiful day!

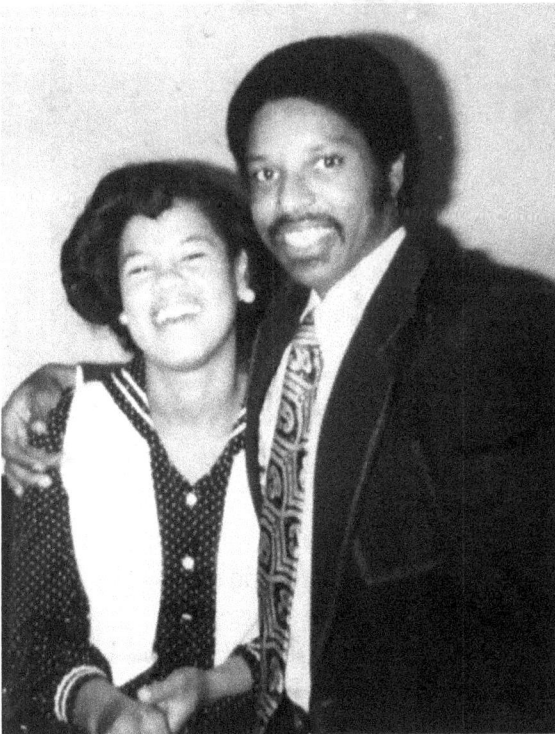

LEFT: Honeymoon, the first stop was Colonial Williamsburg, and later Kill Devil Hills, NC. Our wedding gifts, and my belongings were transported in a van to our home. We walked on the beach a lot and enjoyed great seafood.

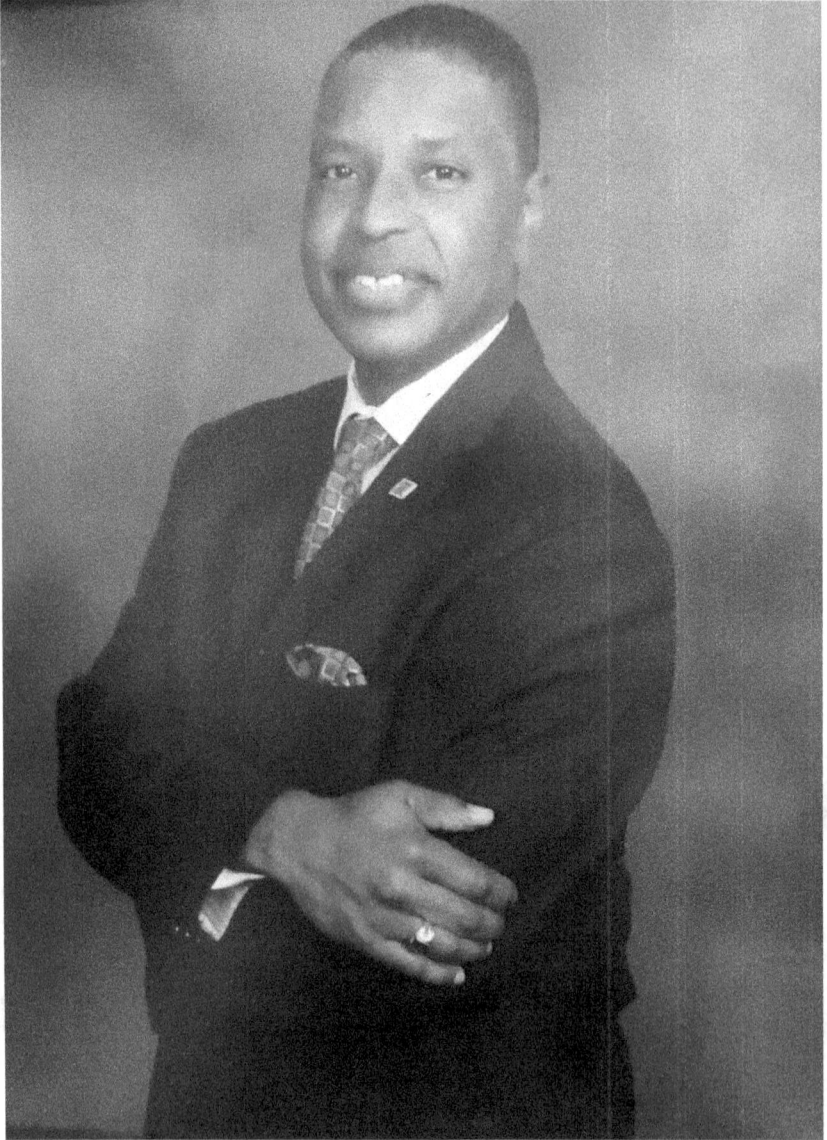

Roy, my husband of 38 years. The kindest and strongest man I know. We cope with differences by allowing each other to be our own person. We often agree to disagree. He is an authentic lover of people and King Jesus. He is the Director of African American Ministries for Texas Baptists.

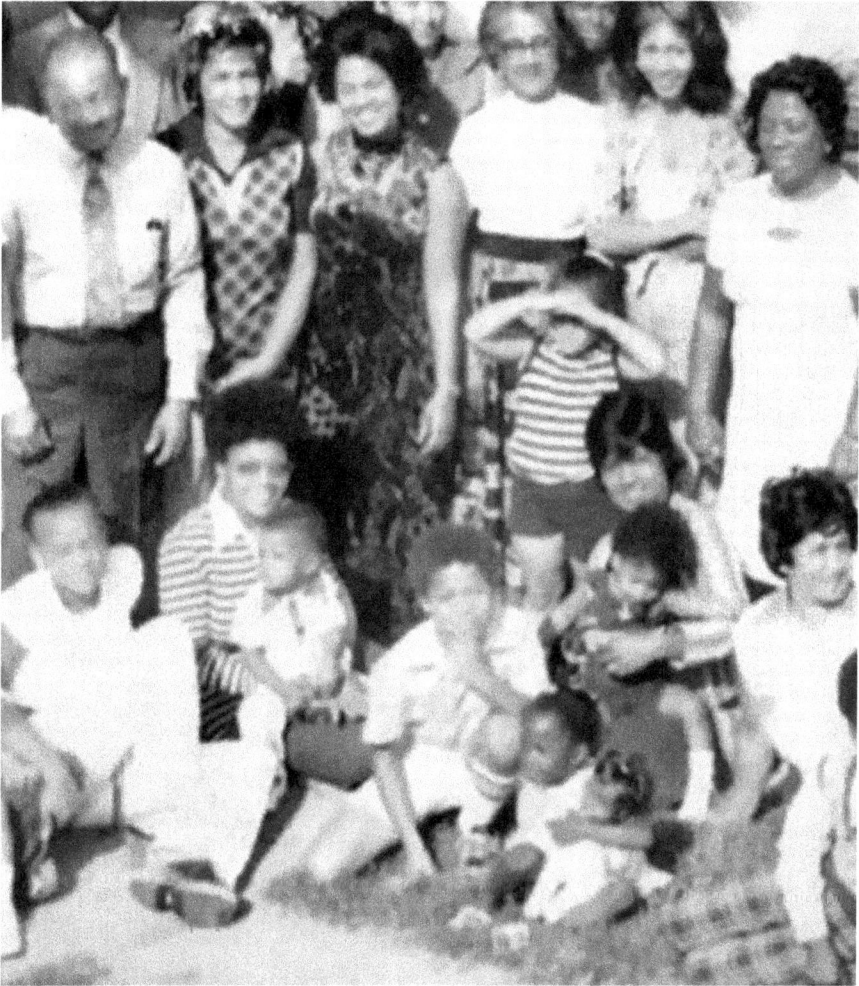

Family reunion in Norfolk, VA. From top left to right: Uncle Dan, my mother's other brother, my sister Jean, Inez, Aunt Bernice, a family friend, and Aunt Evelyn. We were very close to their children, our cousins, Brenda, Sheila, and Yvonne. We also rejoice when we see their children Le'Charn & Kim who lead their lives with promising careers. We also recall our times with uncle Dan's son Anthony.

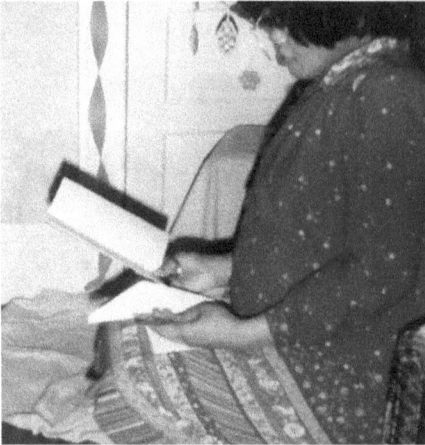

Antepartum mother for our firstborn son, Roy, II. Elmont & Doswell Elementary Schools hosted baby showers by the teachers and one kindergarten class. The Virginia Baptist wives also hosted a shower for us.

Antepartum mother for our second born son, Justin. Roy, II is seated by our next door neighbor's daughter "Ruvette"-p. Virginia Baptists wives hosted a shower for us.

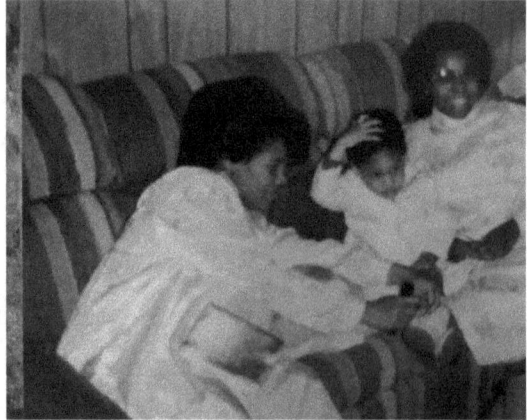

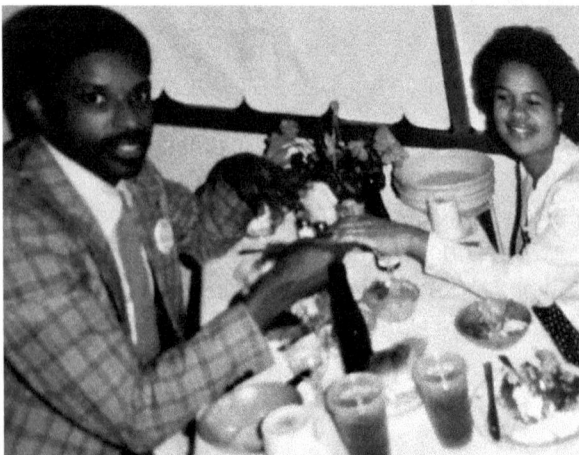

Celebration dinner provided by the hospital after the delivery of Roy II. A unique treat for new parents.

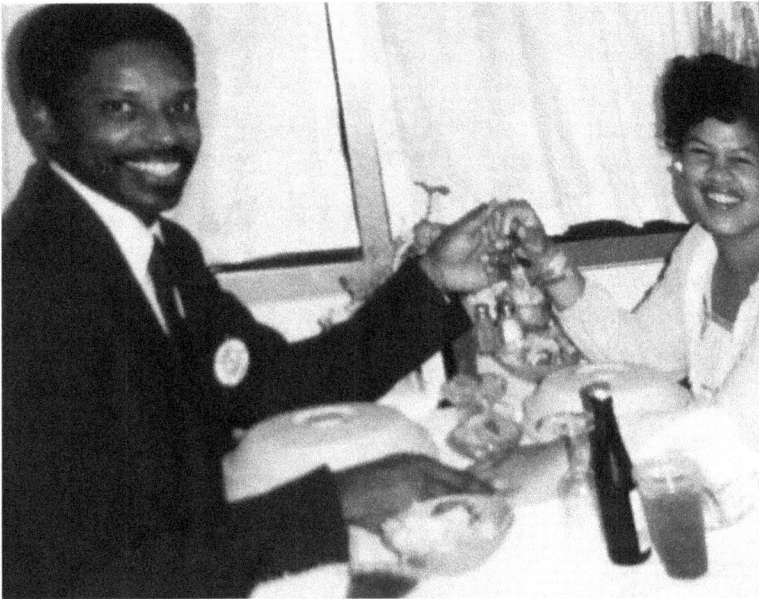

ABOVE: Celebration dinner provided by the hospital for the 50th Anniversary of their healthcare facility. Baby Justin and parents were escorted in a stretch limousine to their home, stopping by the VA Baptist Building for a viewing of the baby.

BELOW: National Baptist Convention attendance. Roy worked with African American Churches at the VA Baptist Building. The family travelled with him across the US when our children were small. We all travelled to Louisville, KY to see Roy receive his Doctor of Ministry Degree at Southern Baptist Theological Seminary.

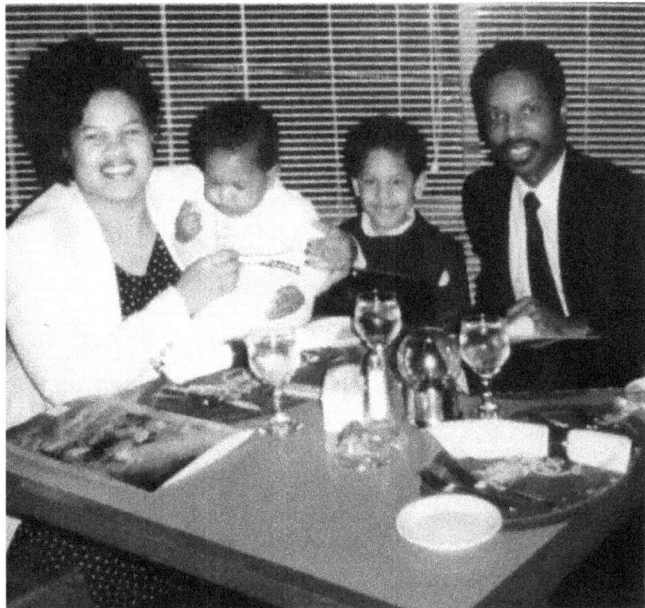

RIGHT: Staying home with the children afforded us many opportunities to visit cultural, entertainment, and educational venues in Henrico and Hanover Counties. They also attended half day pre-k classes at an area church.

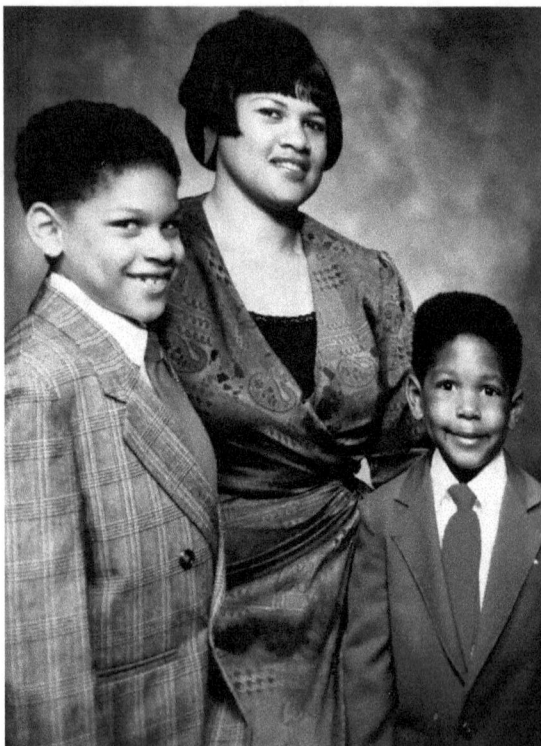

BELOW: "Jay" played football, in Henrico County, Va. He also played for the Youth Choir at our home church, Fifth Street Baptist Church. We moved to Dallas before his high school graduation. Our sons now love Dallas but still miss friends in VA.

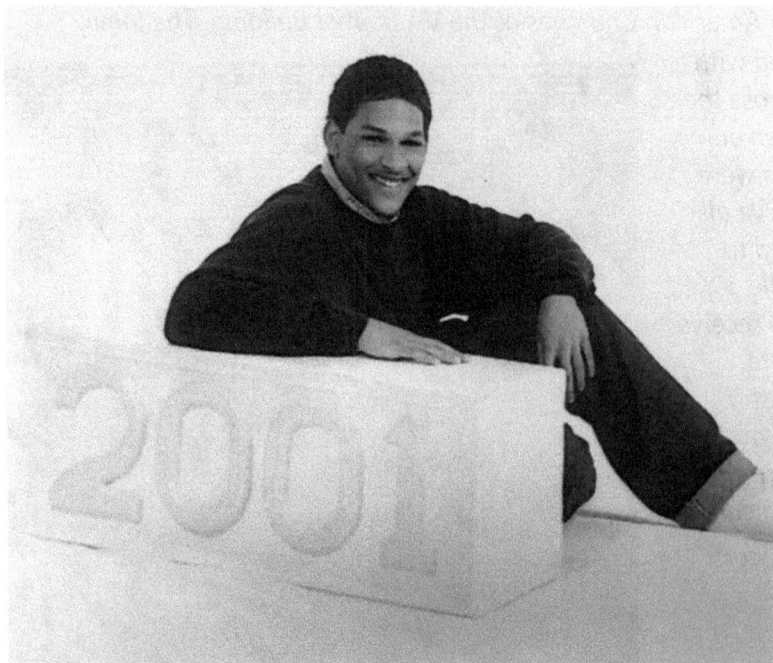

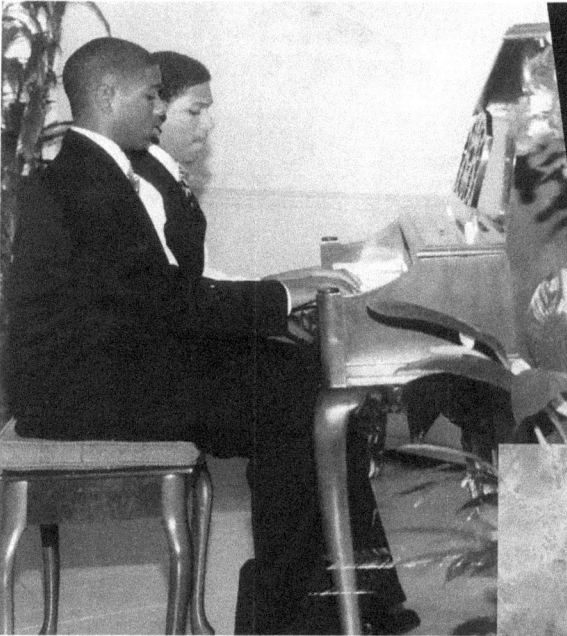

Piano recitals were the order of the day every week in Richmond. I took our sons to every practice as their teachers taught them music theory and other rudiments. They performed in many recitals.

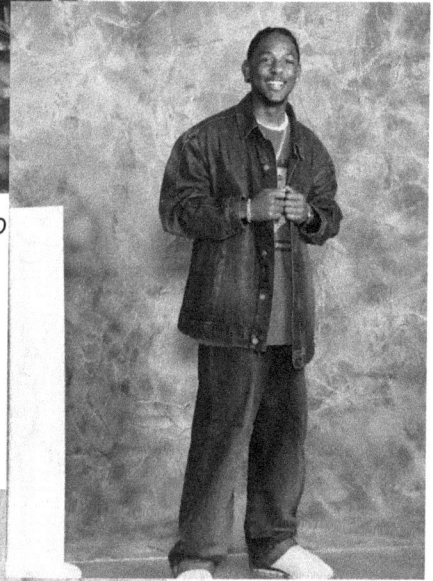

Justin played for the gospel choir and also during many school events. He showed interest in Biology. He also expressed interest in the legal profession and concern for those who could not speak for themselves. His present employment reflects that same care of others.

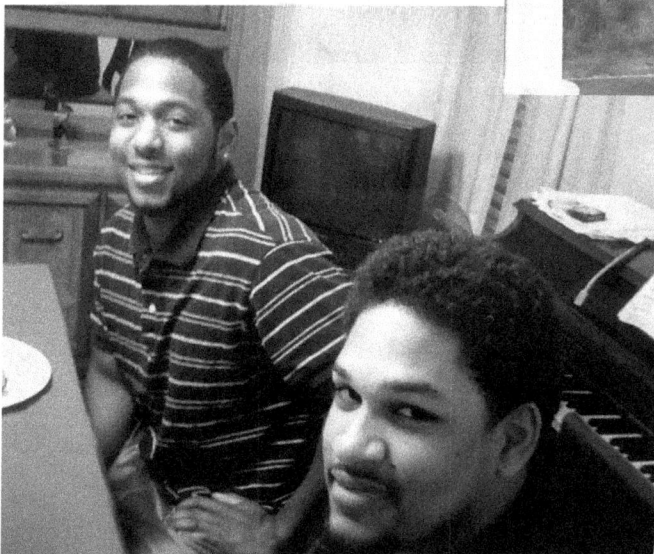

Both sons had a great sense of humor. Both seemed to enjoy high school. They both played the piano in a variety of churches and seemed to develop Christian leadership and grew strong business professionalism.

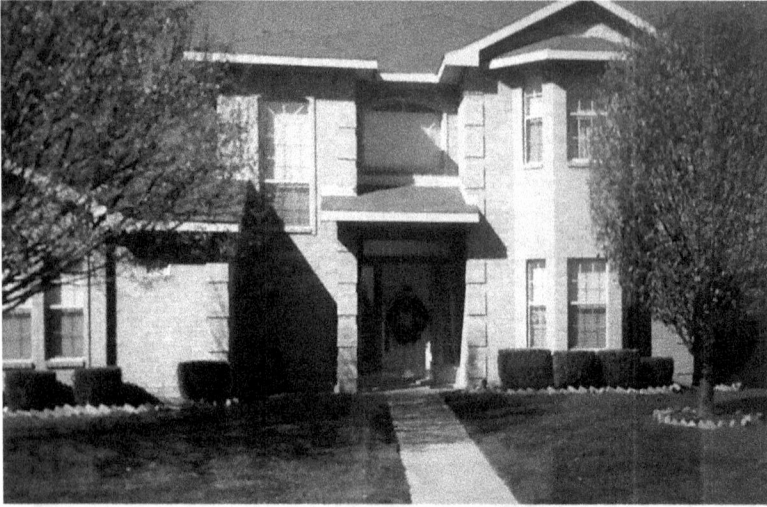

ABOVE: Our home in Texas.
This has been the setting for our
son's gospel choir rehearsals and
the place for piano practices. As
it was in Richmond our home is
a place for family gatherings.

RIGHT: Phil & Thelma are Roy
II's godparents. Our families
have shared compassion for one
another through family & friend
bereavement & healthcare
experiences.

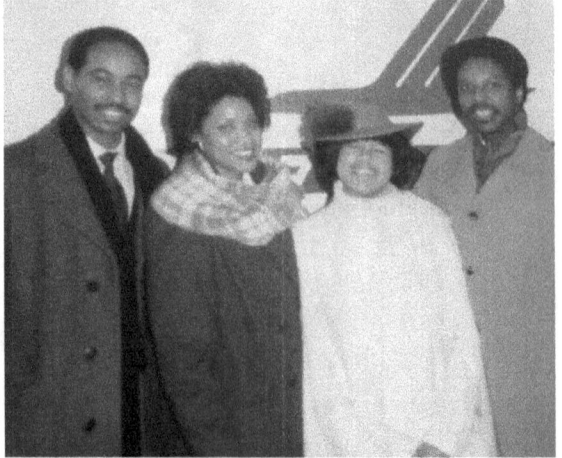

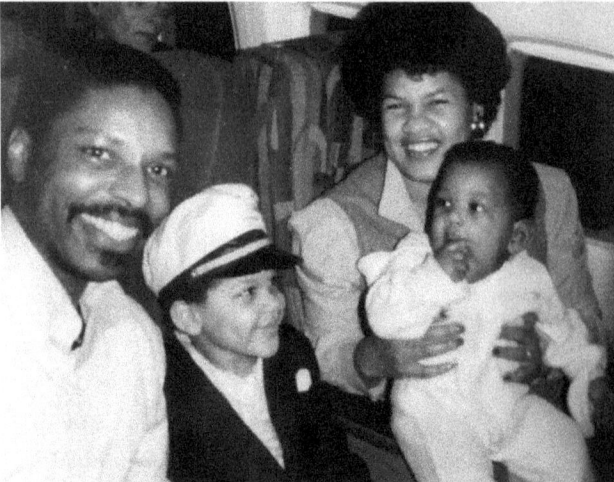

First Plane Trip
to Dallas from
Richmond

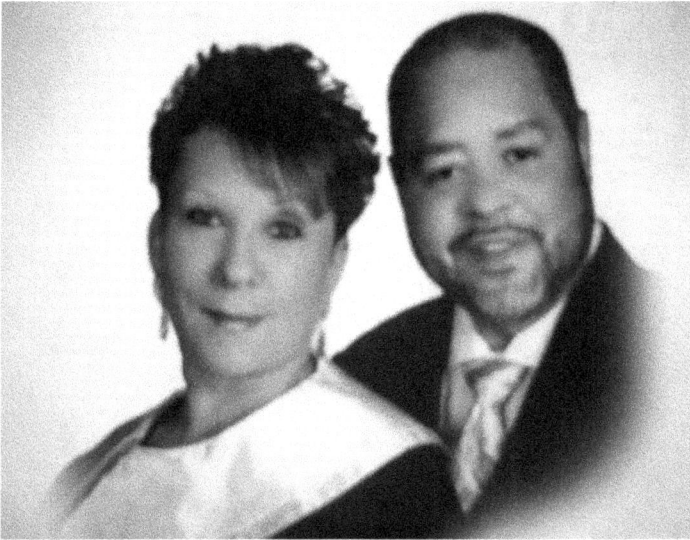

Pastor Todd F. & Mrs. Diane Gray, Fifth Street Baptist Church Richmond, VA.

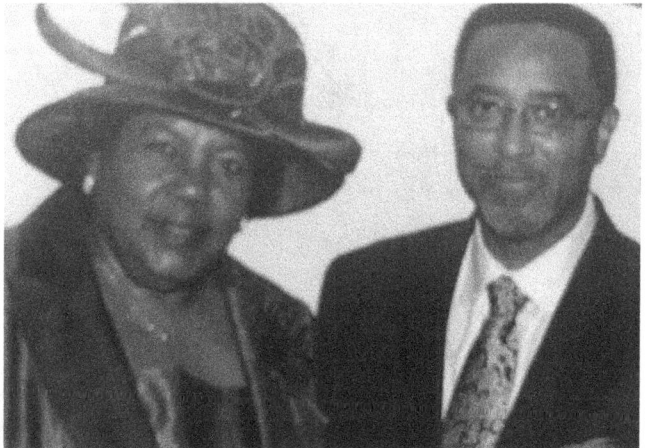

Rev., Dr. Howard & Mrs. Shirley Anderson of The Exciting Singing Hills Baptist Church in Dallas, TX. Pastor & people have walked with us in bereavements and health challenges.

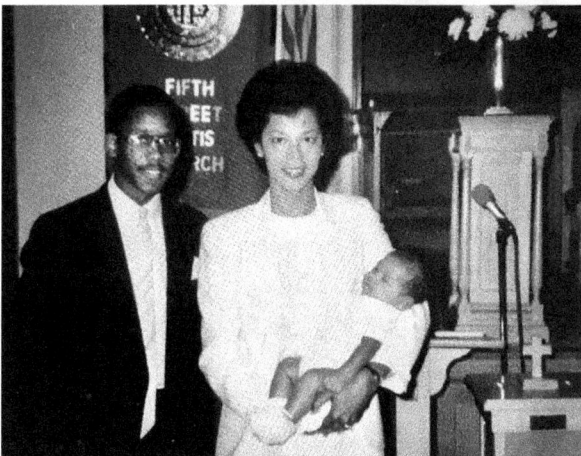

Justin's godparents, Steve & Linda (-p) Malone. Linda was a godly person. We were honored to have them as Justin's godparents.

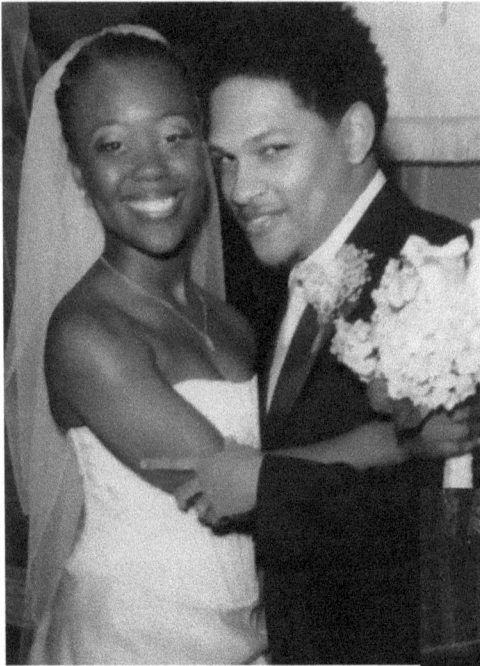

Roy II & Niya's Wedding
Richmond, VA Fifth Street
Baptist Church

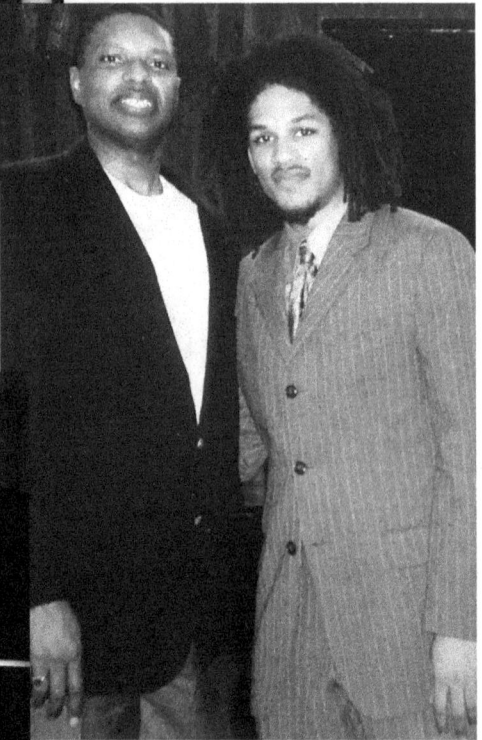

Roy II with father at Senior
Recital at Hampton University

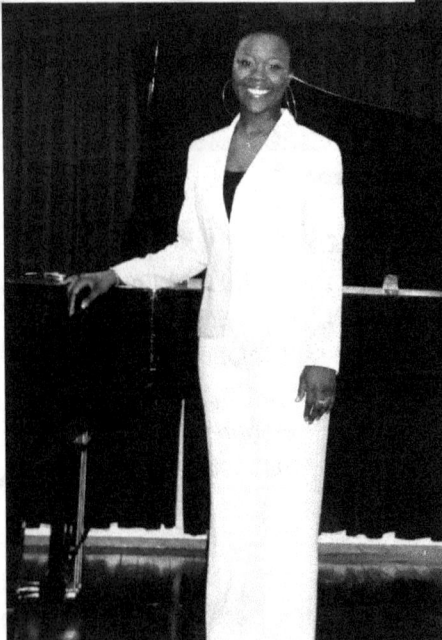

Niya at Hampton University.
Niya has an humble yet strong &
confident way about her. They now
have three children. She is a caring
mother and serves as the Church
Praise and Worship Leader.

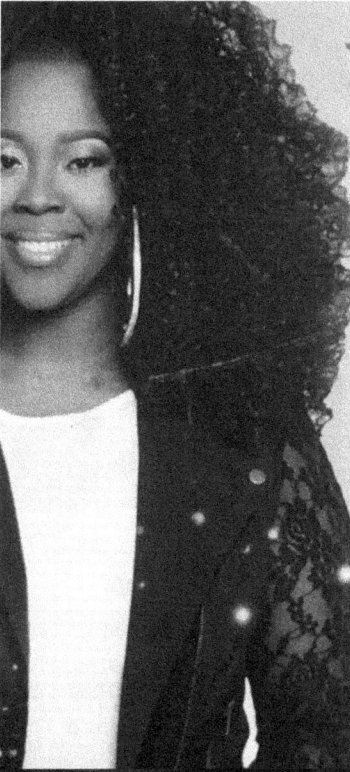

LEFT: A Promotional Photograph from one of Niya's gospel CD's "The Dance"

BELOW: Roy ll is Christian Music Producer, Hymns are his passion, he is a Pianist, Gospel Music Facilitator global ministry pales in comparison to his love for his wife and children. A family man, provider, with a passion for Praise and Worship. "Bring Back the Hymns."

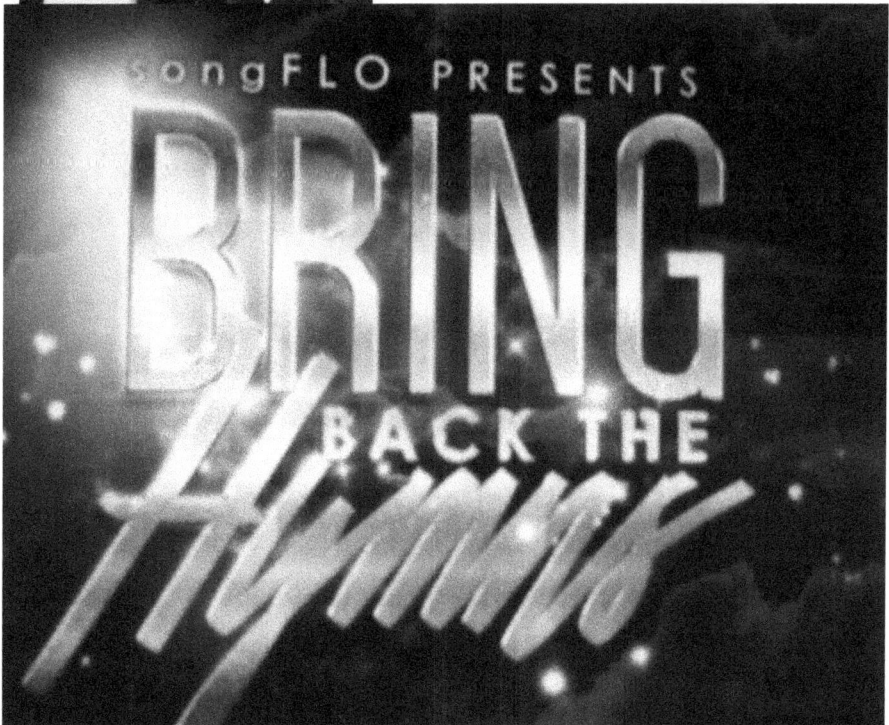

songFLO PRESENTS
BRING
BACK THE
Hymns

RIGHT: Texas Baptist Mission Foundation Cruise to Alaska. Roy sang and played for the devotionals.

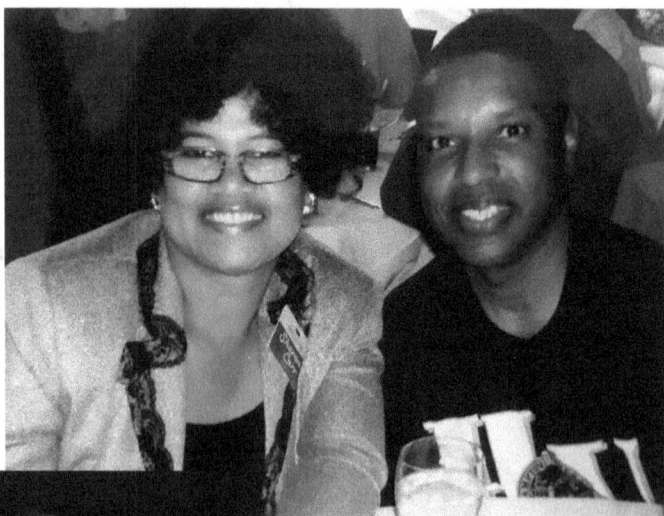

MIDDLE: CenterPointe Baptist Church was sponsored by Texas Baptists and was

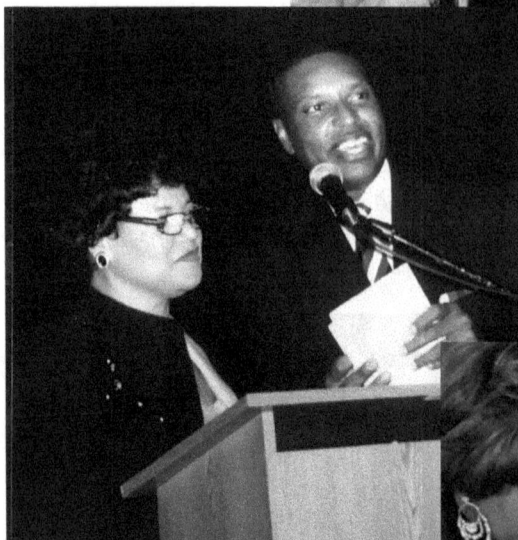

BELOW: Signing the marriage license after performing a marriage ceremony in Texas

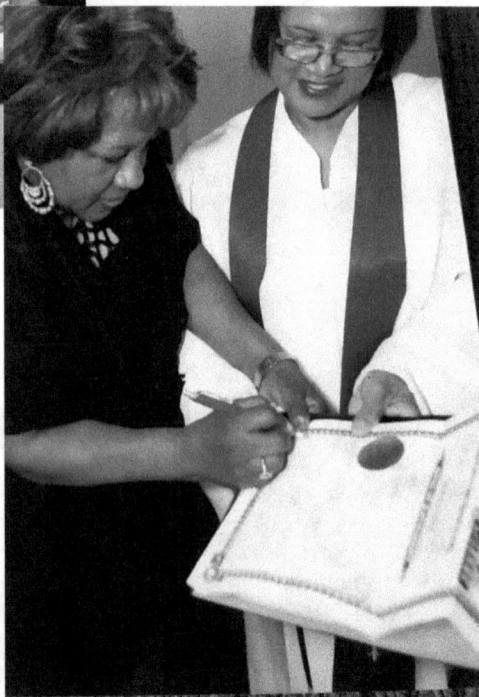

supported by Singing Hills Baptist Church & First Baptist Church in Waxahachie. The work was hard but exhilarating. It was a Church Start in Red Oak, TX. I was given opportunities to preach & teach the gospel message, teach Sunday School, lead the youth ministry and served as the PowerPoint engineer. The church is now in Desoto, TX. Roy is now Pastor Emeritus.

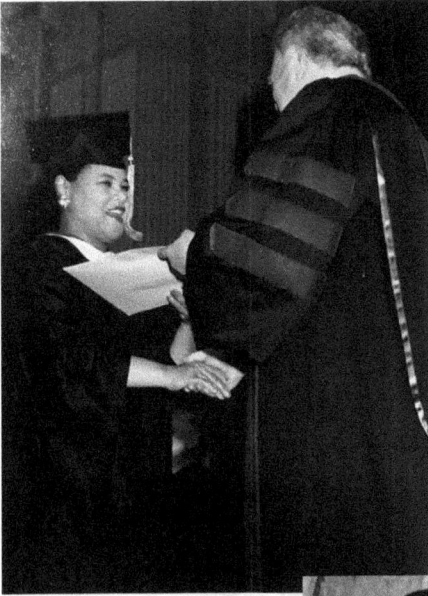

Graduation at Southwestern Baptist Theological Seminary in Fort Worth, TX, from this School of Educational Ministries in Communications, 2004.

A photograph, compliments from the couple whose marriage ceremony I had just performed in Dallas, TX.

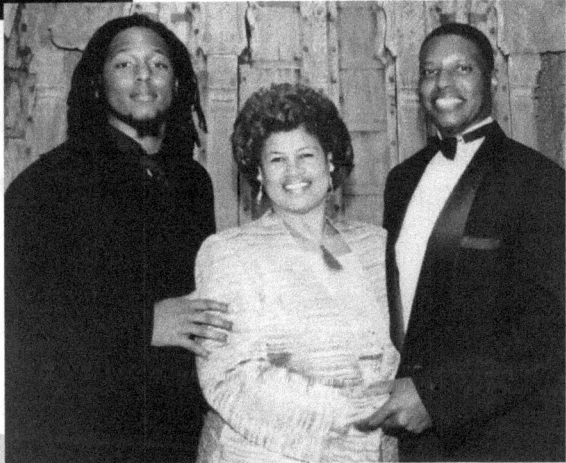

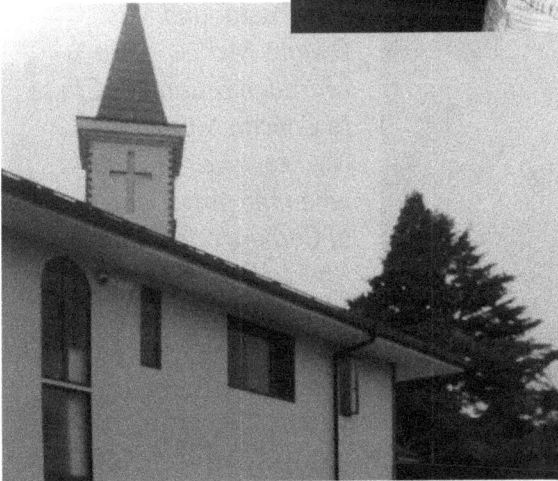

Church in Japan. This short-term mission trip was sponsored by Rev. Charlie Singleton and Texas Baptists African American Ministries. Churches from TX formed a gospel choir. We sang in several churches and other public events.

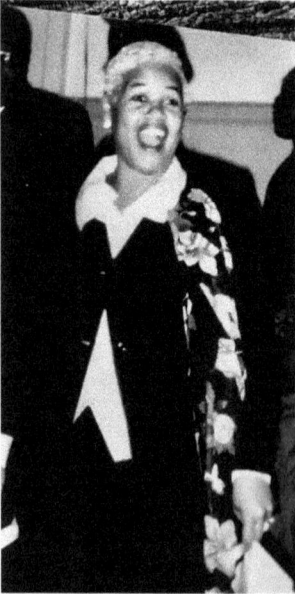

Licensed and ordained at Fifth Street Baptist Church in Richmond, VA. Pastor Gray and our church family were a blessing to me.

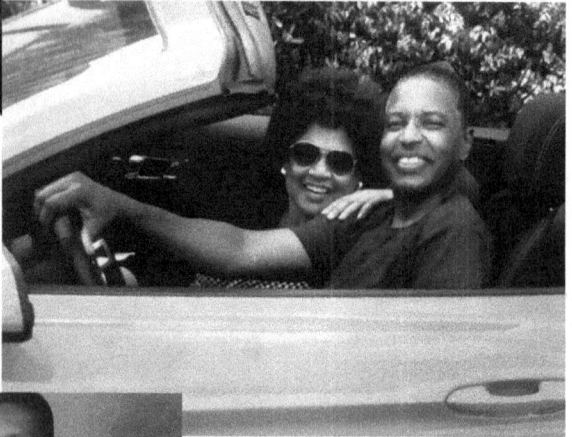

Celebrating in Orlando, Fl after completing the requirements for Board Certification at the Association of Professional Chaplains Conference.

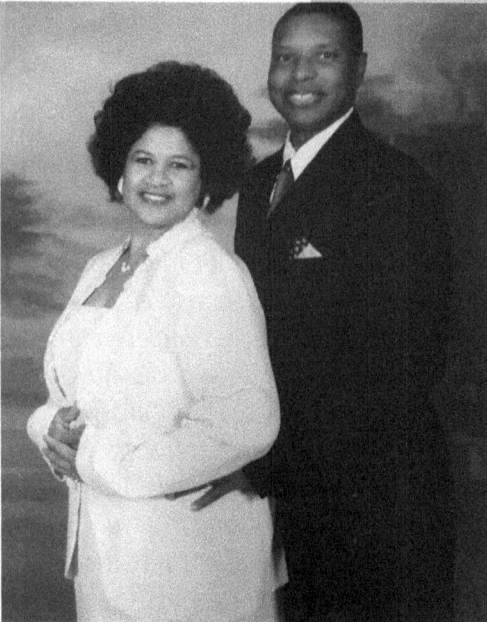

Roy and I facilitated along with Pastor and Mrs. Dwight McKissic at a Marriage & Couples Cruise to Cancun & Cozumel, Mexico. I was grateful when the pastor and people of Cornerstone Baptist Church helped me by granting my acceptance into Southwestern Baptist Theological Seminary in Fort Worth, TX.

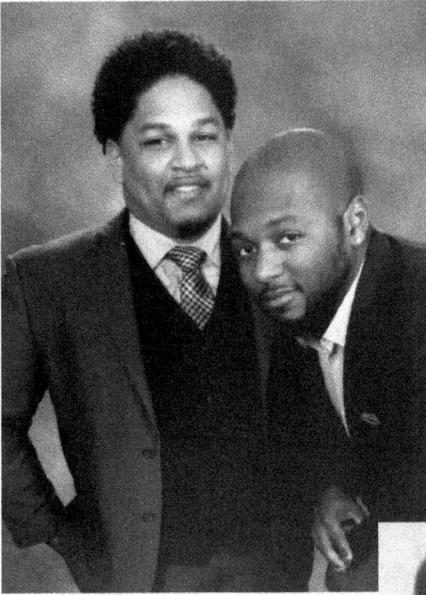

I am and we are ecstatic about how our godly sons "Jay" & Justin have embraced their love for Christ, their churches and their families. They are also great fathers.

Our nieces came from NJ (Alison), DC (Hollis), Houston, TX (Joy), and my youngest sister Jessie-p, among other co-workers, church members and friends to witness my doctoral degree ceremony.

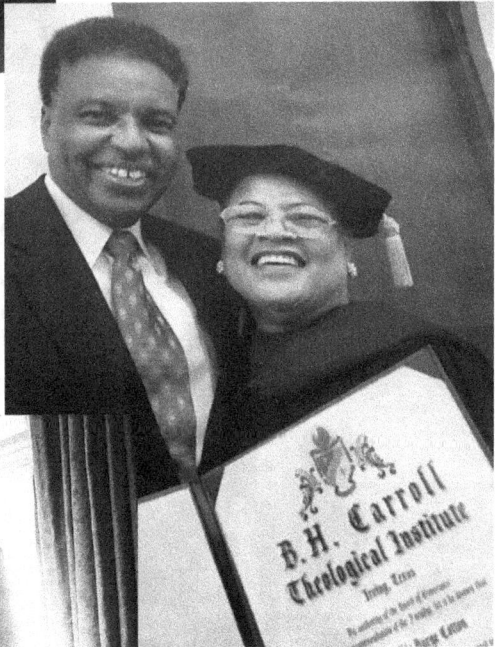

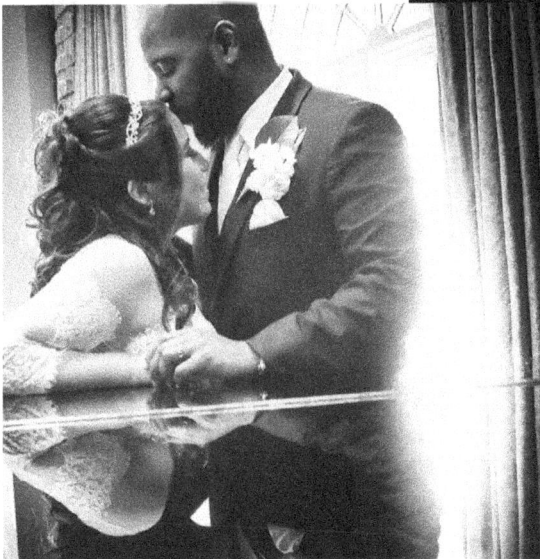

Justin & Carolina's Marriage Ceremony took place at Dallas Baptist University (DBU) They both attended DBU at different times.

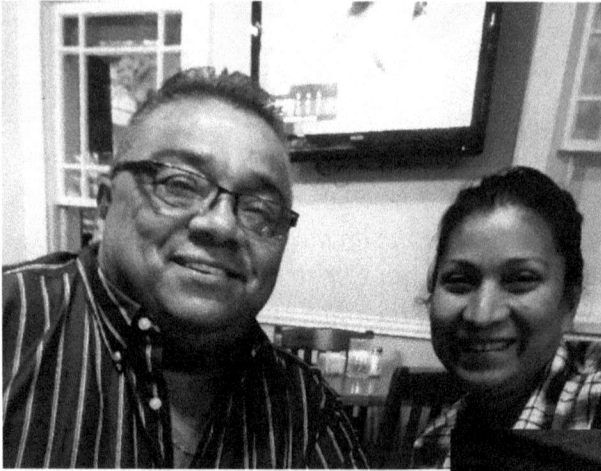

The Avilas, Carolina & Family are warm, and our families have blended well. We seem to have known one another for a long time.

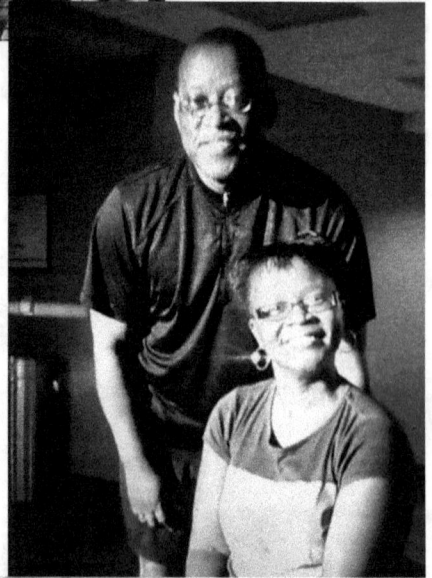

Niya's parents, the Powells from Sacramento, CA. Godly couple with a zest for life. Wonderful grandparents. It seems we have known them for years.

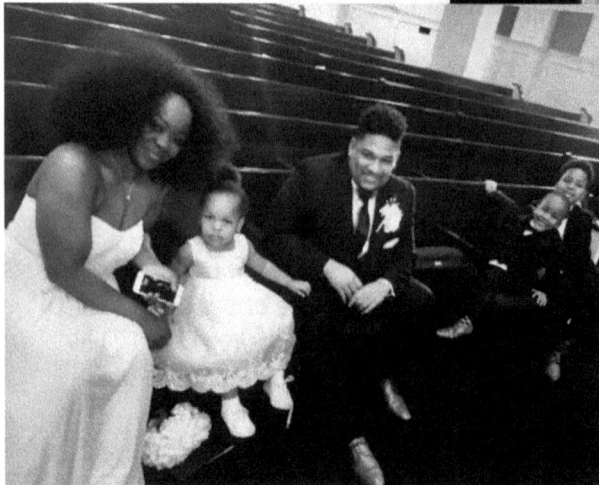

"Jay,"Niya & our grandchildren, Nyla, Eric, & "Rocco, just after Justin and Carolina's Wedding.

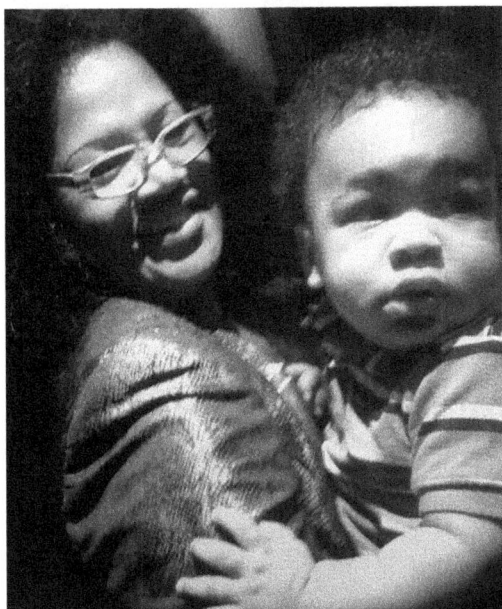

First grandchild, now 8, "Rocco." Heavenly feeling

Second grandchild, Eric. It felt equally amazing for us, Gigi and G-Pop, their grandparents.

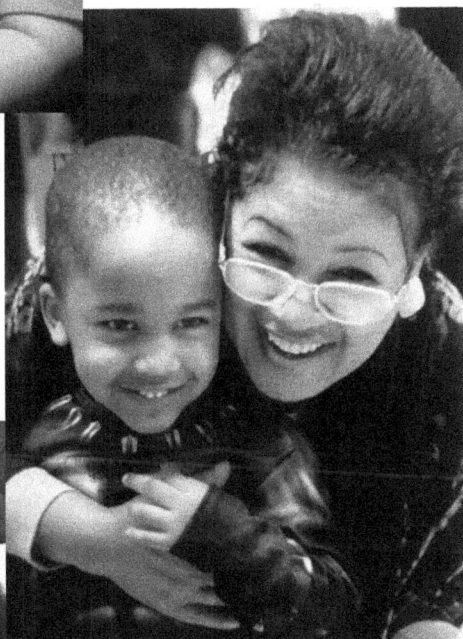

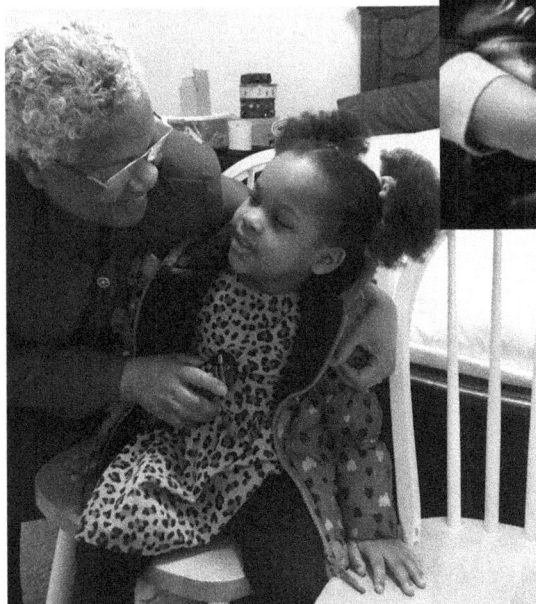

Third grandchild Nyla. We finally have a girl. We felt so blessed.

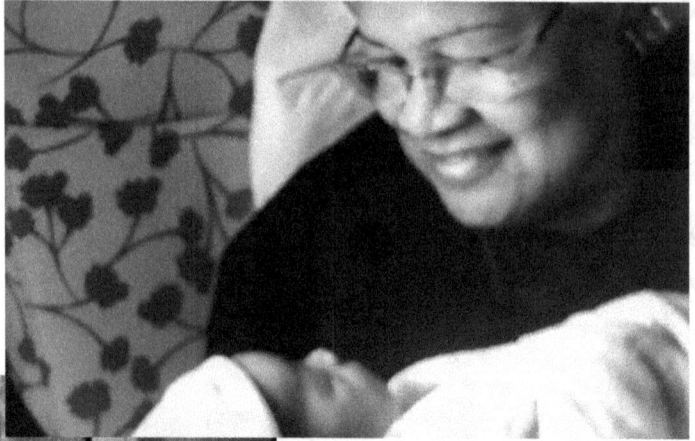

ABOVE: Our fourth grandchild, Justin and Carolina's first child, "JJ." We continue to "melt," just as we did with Jay and Niya's 3 children.

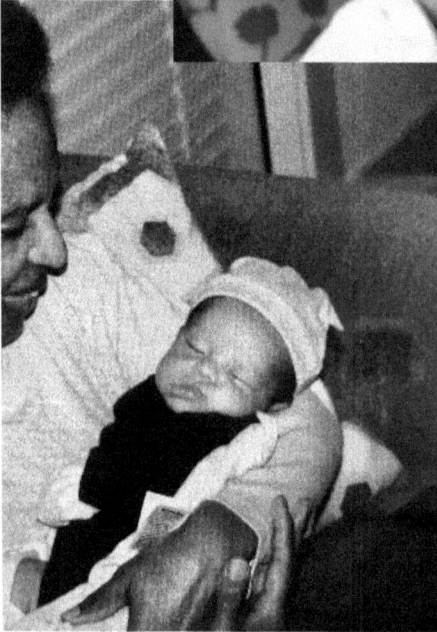

LEFT: I have always loved the way "grandpa" Cotton holds his infant grandchildren.

"JJ," one day old in this photograph. Carolina, Justin's wife, is already a great mother and is also a School Teacher in Midlothian, TX. She is kind with an engaging Christian strength.

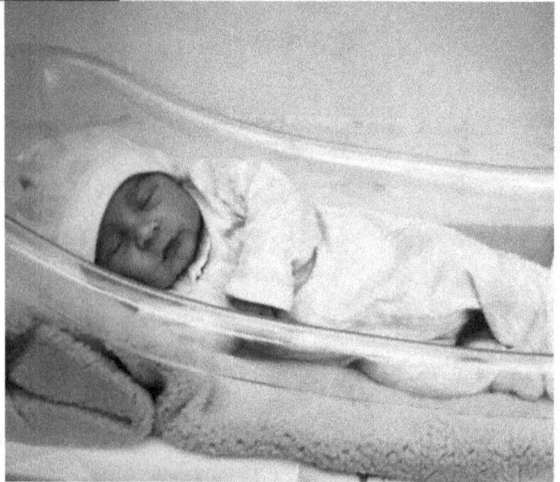

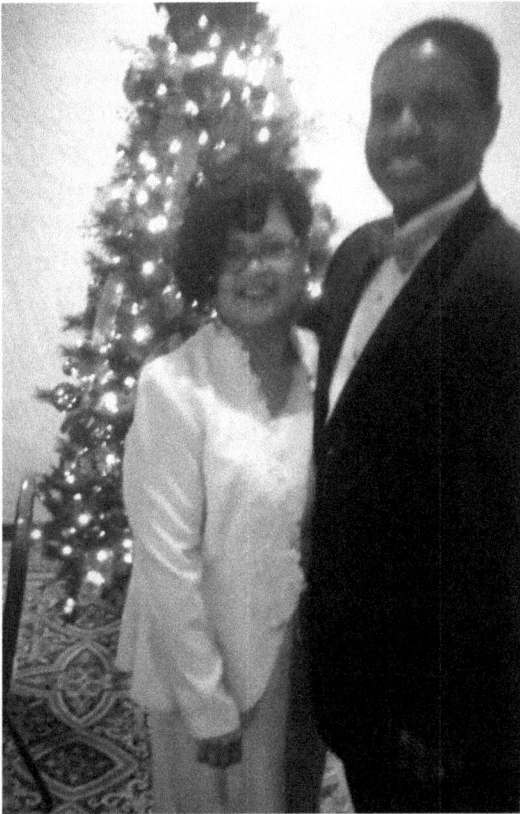

LEFT: Dallas Baptist University Annual Christmas Banquets. The Dallas Baptist Association, and other Texas Baptist events keep all connected to the local and global needs of our communities and beyond.

BELOW: From left to right: Cousin Hobsy from Annapolis,MD. We all spent summers visiting the family. Aunt Callie-p is her mother. Bernice and son Sheldon also live in Annapolis, MD.

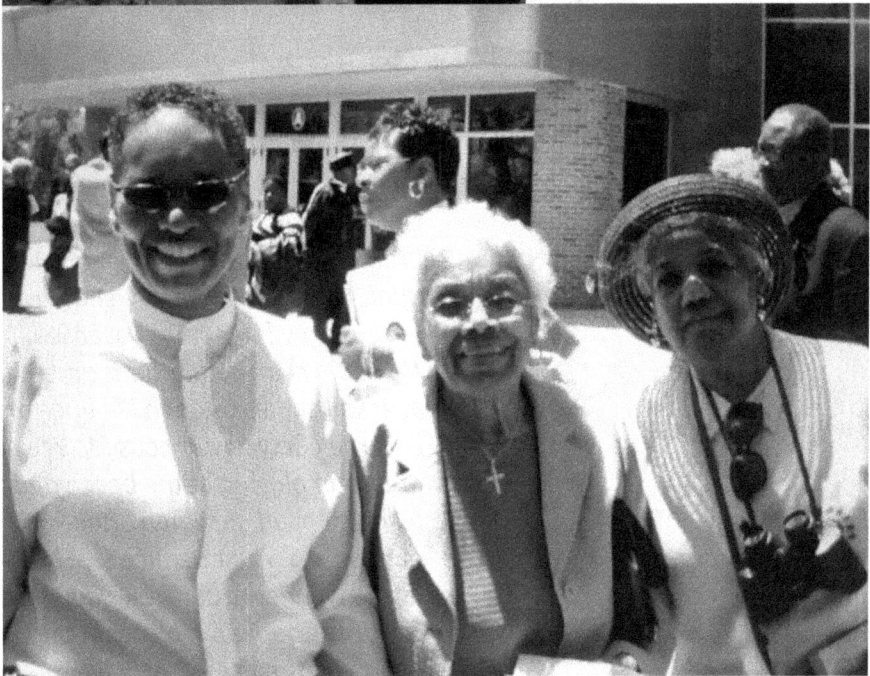

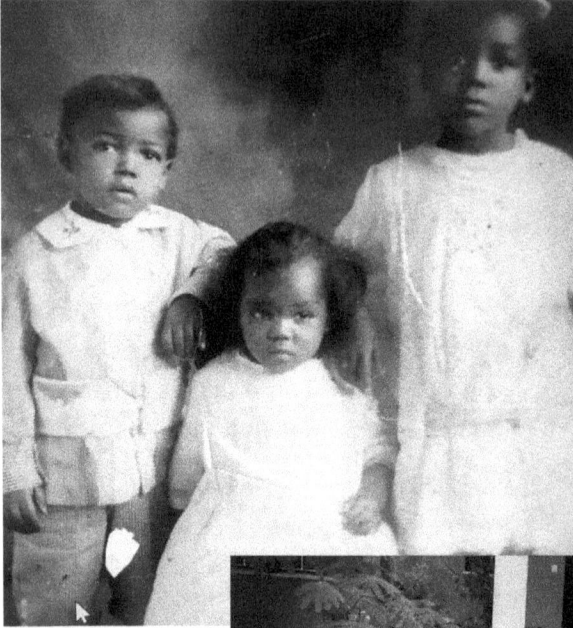

A photograph cousin Hobsy gave to me of my dad, John-p, Aunt Callie-p, & Aunt Lou-p, all born in Annapolis, MD. Their dad, Cicero-p was in the Navy.

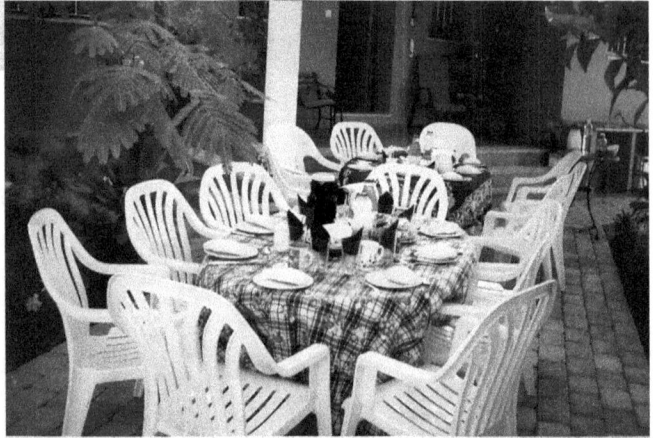

Denia, Spain-Short Term Mission Trip. I was given the opportunity to provide my testimony in entry level Spanish.

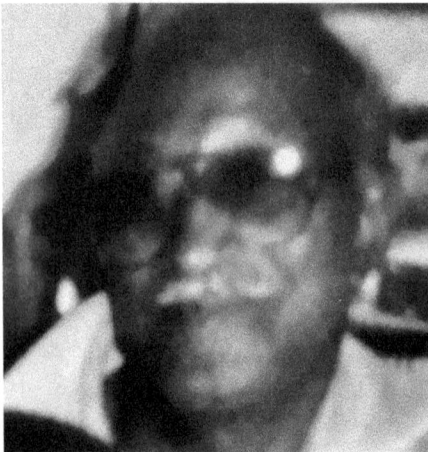

Uncle Mike -p, was my mother's brother & Aretha-p, our beautiful aunt. He stood in at my wedding because my father was deceased. He had a calm caring spirit and that love still shines through Maurice and Laverne (Calvin) our cousins. We had great fun playing at the beach and fellowshipped at church often with our cousins. Aunt Bernice (-p) was also a wonderful aunt. Her daughter Sandra (Charles), is also a great and caring cousin in Indianapolis, IN.

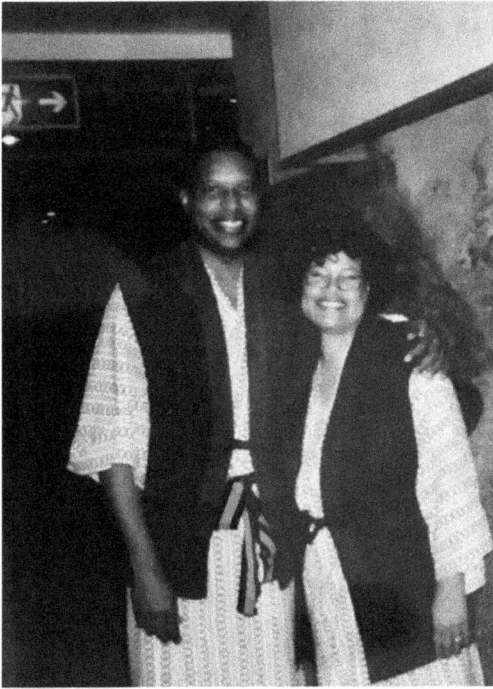

Gospel Choir sang in Japan on a short- term mission trip. The choir was formed from African American choir members from all over the state of Texas. We were a hit in Jesus' Name!

Undergraduate degree. Bachelor of Fine Arts in Art Education. Daddy passed away just before graduation. I felt dad's presence there.

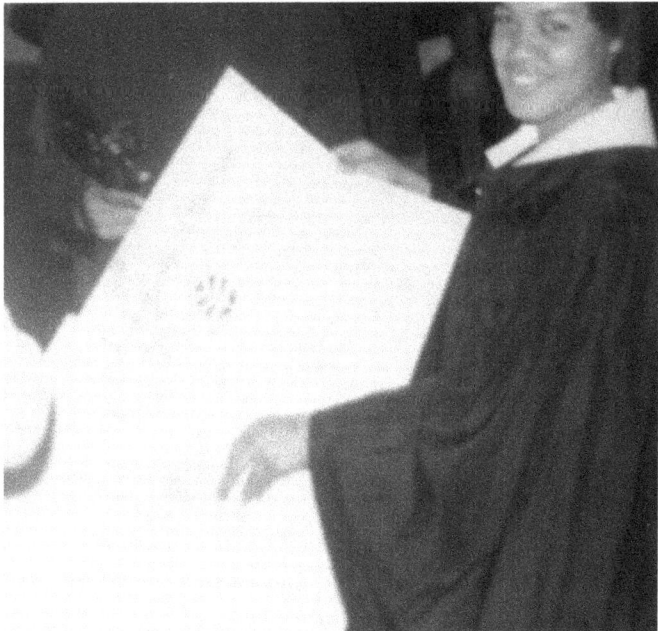

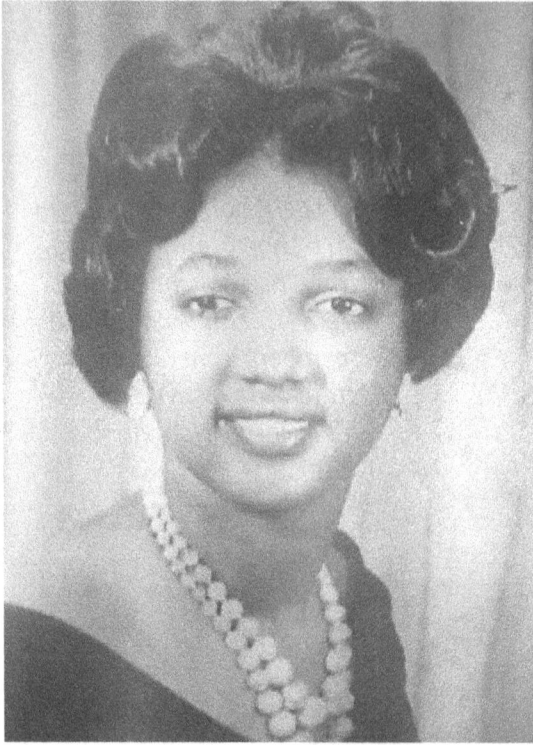

Cousin Sandra (Charles) is very close to the sisters. Their children Charles, Jr. and Monica have kept up their parents professionalism in their careers.

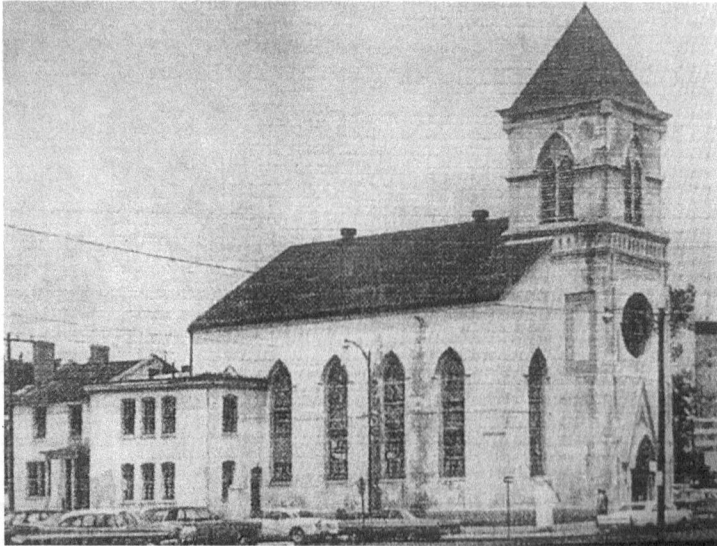

Bank Street Baptist Church in Norfolk, VA. I made a profession of faith here. I sang in the youth choir and loved visiting the sick & "shut-in" during Youth Week every summer.

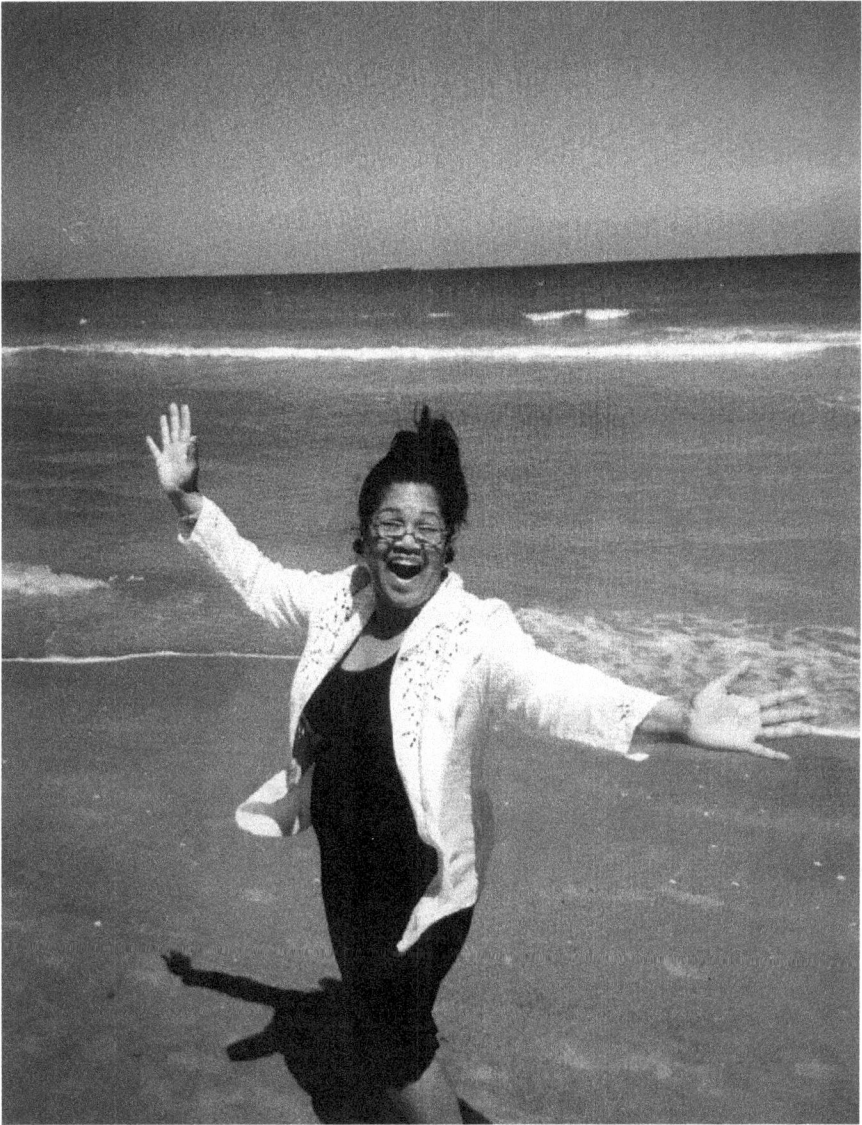

Celebration! What an exciting journey this has been. I experienced unexpected surprises, renewed revelations, but most of all spiritual healing with the writing of this book with photographs. We wanted the patients in our study to back track and recall notable people and experiences that would help them to "re-see" their lives despite difficult circumstances. It is my prayer that you will spread this kind of interpersonal hope in your own lives as well as the unique population of antepartum women in the 21st century.

www.ingramcontent.com/pod-product-compliance
Lightning Source LLC
Chambersburg PA
CBHW072242270326
41930CB00010B/2240